DEBATES IN PERSONALISATION

Edited by
Catherine Needham and Jon Glasby

P

First published in Great Britain in 2014 by

Policy Press
University of Bristol
1-9 Old Park Hill
Clifton
Bristol BS2 8BB
UK
t: +44 (0)117 954 5940
pp-info@bristol.ac.uk
www.policypress.co.uk

North America office:
Policy Press
c/o The University of Chicago Press
1427 East 60th Street
Chicago, IL 60637, USA
t: +1 773 702 7700
f: +1 773 702 9756
sales@press.uchicago.edu
www.press.uchicago.edu

© Policy Press 2014

British Library Cataloguing in Publication Data
A catalogue record for this book is available from the British Library

Library of Congress Cataloging-in-Publication Data
A catalog record for this book has been requested

ISBN 978 1 44731 342 7 paperback

The right of Catherine Needham and Jon Glasby to be identified as editors of this work has
been asserted by them in accordance with the Copyright, Designs and Patents Act 1988.

Cover design by Policy Press
Front cover: www.shutterstock.com
Printed and bound by CPI Group (UK) Ltd, Croydon, CR0 4YY
Policy Press uses environmentally responsible print partners

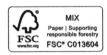

Contents

Part Five: Responses and conclusions

List of tables and figures

Table

Figures

Notes on contributors

Vidhya Alakeson is deputy chief executive at the Resolution Foundation, an independent think tank. She is also a leading consultant and internationally recognised expert in the personalisation of health and social care. She is the mental health lead for the personal health budgets delivery programme at NHS England and has also been closely involved in the development of personalisation in the American Medicaid programme. She is the author of *Delivering personal health budgets: A guide to policy and practice* (Policy Press, 2014). Vidhya previously worked for the US Department of Health and Human Services and before that, for the UK Treasury and Prime Minister's Strategy Unit.

Peter Beresford OBE is professor of social policy and director of the Centre for Citizen Participation at Brunel University. He is a long-term user of mental health services and chair of Shaping Our Lives, the user-controlled and disabled people's organisation and network. He has a longstanding involvement in issues of participation as an activist, educator, researcher and writer. He is co-author of *Supporting people: Towards person-centred support* (2011, Policy Press) and *Personalisation*, (2014, Policy Press).

Christine Bond In 1998 Christine gained a BA (Hons) in business studies (hotel and catering management); during this time she became physically disabled and found it hard to pursue a career in the industry. After completing this course she worked in the disability movement, first as an administrator then later also becoming a disability equality trainer. After moving to Norfolk she continued to be involved in the disability movement and worked for community services where she supported disabled people. She has also supported a self advocacy group for people with learning difficulties. Christine strongly believes in the social model of disability and fighting for people's rights.

Jenni Brooks has been a research fellow at the Social Policy Research Unit, University of York, since 2010. During this time she has worked on a variety of projects around different aspects of the personalisation of social care. Projects have explored the needs of, and support available for, people with complex needs, family carers, physically disabled young adults and people living with dementia. Her research interests include the role of music in dementia care and the development of the social care workforce, particularly the role of personal assistants.

Sarah Carr is an independent mental health and social care knowledge consultant. She is an honorary visiting fellow at the School of Social Policy and Social Work (University of York), honorary senior lecturer at the School of Social Policy (University of Birmingham), a fellow of the Royal Society of Arts, co-vice chair of the National Survivor User Network and a member of the editorial board of *Disability and Society*. Previously she was a senior research analyst at the Social Care Institute for Excellence. Sarah has a particular interest in mental health. She also has lived experience.

Simon Duffy is director of The Centre for Welfare Reform. Simon is a philosopher and social activist who works to redesign the welfare system to promote citizenship for all. He led the development of self-directed support, for which he was awarded the RSA's 2008 Prince Albert Medal, and the SPA's 2011 Award for Outstanding Contribution to Social Policy. He has been a Harkness Fellow and has a PhD in moral philosophy. Simon is chair of the Housing and Support Alliance, policy adviser to the Campaign for a Fair Society and an honorary senior research fellow at the University of Birmingham.

Julien Forder is the director of the Personal Social Services Research Unit, University of Kent, and a principal research fellow at the London School of Economics and Political Science. Julien was the principal investigator for the Department of Health-funded evaluation of the personal health budget pilot programme. The national evaluation began in 2009 and a final report was published in November 2012.

Jon Glasby is professor of health and social care and director of the Health Services Management Centre at the University of Birmingham. Specialising in joint working between health and social care, Jon is involved in regular policy analysis and advice. He is the author of a series of leading textbooks on health and social services, sits on the advisory board of Policy Press, and is editor-in-chief of the *Journal of Integrated Care*. He is currently a non-executive director of the Birmingham Children's Hospital and, from 2003 to 2009, was the Secretary of State's representative on the board of the UK Social Care Institute for Excellence.

Caroline Glendinning is emeritus professor of social policy in the Social Policy Research Unit at the University of York. Her research interests include social and health care services, disability, family care and comparative studies of long-term care funding, organisation and delivery.

Victoria Hart is a registered social worker who has worked in learning disabilities services, older adults services and in specialist older adults mental health services. She now works for the Care Quality Commission as an inspector.

Melanie Henwood OBE is an independent health and social care research consultant. Between 2002 and 2010 she was a lay member of the General Social Care Council, and was vice chair from 2008. Melanie has held specialist adviser roles to the House of Commons Health Select Committee, the MS Society and the Joseph Rowntree Foundation. Previously Melanie has held visiting fellowships at the London School of Economics and Political Science, the University of Leeds, and the University of New South Wales, Australia. She has more than 30 years' experience in research and analysis, focusing particularly on care and support for older people, people with disabilities and their carers.

Karen Jones is a senior research fellow in the Personal Social Services Research Unit at the University of Kent. Karen managed the evaluation of the personal health budget pilot programme and was the principal link to the Department of Health policy team and pilot sites.

Liz Lloyd is reader in social gerontology in the School for Policy Studies at the University of Bristol. She is an experienced researcher in the field of ageing, with a particular interest in older people's experiences of care. Her published outputs focus on the end of life in old age, dignity in care and the ethics of care. She is the author of *Health and care in ageing societies: A new international approach* (Policy Press, 2012). Liz is currently the UK leader of HARP (Healthy Ageing in Residential Places), an international study of promising practices in long-term residential care.

Sian Lockwood OBE is the first chief executive of Community Catalysts, a community interest company launched by NAAPS (now Shared Lives Plus) in January 2010. Over the four years since its launch Community Catalysts has worked with a range of local partners (councils, independent providers and third sector infrastructure organisations) to help local people use their gifts, talents and imagination to set up sustainable social care and health enterprises and to support the development of Shared Lives. Sian was awarded an OBE for services to social care in 2010.

Jill Manthorpe is professor of social work and director of the Social Care Workforce Research Unit at King's College London. The Unit undertakes studies of social care for the Department of Health through investigating new roles, system changes and workforce profiles and setting these in the context of user experience and social care practice. Her work on personalisation has included studies of individual budgets, self-directed support and personalisation in rural areas. Jill has particular interest in adult safeguarding research including studies of adult serious care reviews, the Mental Capacity Act 2005, risk and personalisation, and the Care Act 2014. She is emeritus senior investigator of the National Institute for Health Research.

Wendy Mitchell has been a research fellow in the Social Policy Research Unit at the University of York since 2000. During this time, Wendy has worked on a range of projects exploring the health and social care needs and experiences of disabled and chronically ill people, their carers and other family members. Within this, a number of projects have focused on personalised adult social care, particularly personal budgets, and have involved adults, especially young people with communication and/or cognitive impairments.

Catherine Needham is a reader in public policy and public management at the Health Services Management Centre, University of Birmingham. Her research interests focus on public service reform and policy innovation. She has published a wide range of articles, chapters and books for academic and practitioner audiences, many of them focused on personalisation and personal budgets. Her most recent book is *Personalising public services: Understanding the personalisation agenda* (Policy Press, 2011).

Helga Pile is a national officer in the local government section at UNISON, where she leads on social care for the union. Helga has worked at UNISON since 2006, during which she has served as a Skills for Care board member and a member of the Social Work Task Force.

Colin Royle became a full-time carer to his father, Malcolm, who suffers with early onset dementia, in 2008. After initially struggling to find a suitable package of care, Colin and Malcolm began using a personal health budget in 2009. Colin became extremely passionate about the implementation of personal health budgets and in 2012, co-founded peoplehub, a community interest company that aims to ensure that personal health budgets stay 'true to purpose'. peoplehub now facilitates several peer networks across the country, has helped to develop emerging policy with the Department of Health, and is currently working with NHS England in delivering a national peer leadership programme.

Lucy Series is a research associate at Cardiff Law School. Lucy is currently working on a project funded by the Nuffield Foundation looking at welfare cases in the Court of Protection. Her research interests include legal capacity, disability rights and community care law. Lucy's PhD research at Exeter University examined the Mental Capacity Act 2005 and the deprivation of liberty safeguards. She previously worked at the Centre for Disability Law and Policy at NUI Galway. Prior to her PhD in law, Lucy studied psychology and philosophy and worked in a variety of roles in health and social care.

Colin Slasberg qualified as a social worker in the 1970s with a career spanning practice, operational management and strategic planning in both adults and children's services, serving urban and rural communities and working in shire and unitary councils. He currently works independently, focusing on the development of policy and practice to deliver personalised supports within the context of the need to find new ways to manage the political and legal tensions between needs and resources. In addition to working on a consultancy basis, he has had a number of papers published that address this theme.

Part One
Introduction and overview

ONE

Introduction:
debating personalisation

Catherine Needham and Jon Glasby

For anyone working in or receiving adult social care services, the personalisation agenda is of fundamental importance. Different people may love it or loathe it – may be fully supportive, completely opposed and/or just confused – but the shifts in policy and practice that personalisation might imply are potentially far-reaching and certainly hard to ignore. Of all the changes that have taken place in adult social care (and increasingly in other sectors too), it is personalisation that stands out as one of the key themes of the past decade, and quite possibly as one of the key agendas of the next ten years.

Under New Labour, the government's *Putting People First* concordat pledged to achieve a 'system-wide transformation' in which people using services have 'maximum choice, control and power over the support services they receive' (DH, 2007, pp 2-3) and in which personal budgets are available 'for everyone eligible for publicly funded adult social care support other than in circumstances where people require emergency access to provision'. Acknowledging the role of organisations such as In Control (see below) and a number of cutting-edge voluntary organisations and local authorities, the government recognised the importance of local and national leadership to help support and build on 'the first stage in a unique attempt to co-produce, co-develop and co-evaluate a major public service reform' (DH, 2007, p 5). Similar sentiments have also been expressed by the coalition government in *A vision for adult social care* (DH, 2010a, p 15):

> Our vision starts with securing the best outcomes for people. People, not service providers or systems, should hold the choice and control about their care. Personal budgets and direct payments are a powerful way to give people control. Care is a uniquely personal service. It supports people at their most vulnerable, and often covers the most intimate

and private aspects of their lives. With choice and control, people's dignity and freedom is protected and their quality of life is enhanced. Our vision is to make sure everyone can get the personalised support they deserve.

Building on this, one of seven key principles of *A vision for adult social care* was 'personalisation', described as an approach in which:

> Individuals not institutions take control of their care. Personal budgets, preferably as direct payments, are provided to all eligible people. Information about care and support is available for all local people, regardless of whether or not they fund their own care. (DH, 2010a, p 8)

As we explain in Chapter Two of this book, the concept of personalisation is broadly (and often poorly) defined, but two key mechanisms include:

- *Direct payments* (cash payments to disabled people in lieu of directly provided services). Pioneered by disabled people themselves, direct payments emerged informally in different localities in the mid-1980s and were formally introduced under 1996 legislation after sustained campaigning by disabled people's organisations.
- *Personal budgets* (developed initially by a social enterprise known as In Control and subsequently incorporated into official policy at pace and scale). In one sense, a personal budget is nothing more complicated than trying to be up front with people from day one about how much money is available to spend on meeting their needs, and then allowing them a say over how the money is spent (with one option being a direct payment, but with other options as well for how the money is managed).

From the beginning, personalisation has been the subject of significant debate and controversy. Approaching the issues from different standpoints and perspectives, different commentators have seen personalisation either as a radical revolution in which services are transformed and power shifted dramatically in favour of people using services or an attempt to roll back the boundaries of the welfare state, undermine public sector services and pass off state responsibilities onto people already in need. As the implications of personalisation have started to become clearer over time, key questions have included the following:

- Is personalisation transferring risk and responsibility from the state to the individual – or is it promoting more of a partnership of equals in which risk is shared in a positive way by the individual and the system together?
- Is personalisation connecting people more fully with their family, friends and communities – or is it closing down collective spaces such as day centres and isolating people in their homes?
- Can personalisation work equally well for all types of people using services – and in particular for older people?
- Will personalisation free people up to choose what sort of relationship they want with their friends and families – or will it place an unacceptable burden on unpaid women carers?
- How can the positive approaches to risk inherent in personalisation be reconciled with safeguarding?
- Will personalisation deepen inequalities between people using social care services – or more fully tailor responses to individual need so that outcomes are more equal?
- Is personalisation de-professionalising social workers and depressing terms and conditions for the broader social care workforce – or will it lead to a return to the values of community social work and to better relationships between care workers and their employers?
- Is personalisation adding to bureaucracy and legal ambiguity – or is it simplifying people's entitlement to resources?
- Is personalisation a concept that could revolutionise other areas of the welfare state – or is it being stretched into other sectors (such as health) on the basis of a weak evidence base?

Depending on where you sit, personalisation is either the best thing since sliced bread or the end of the welfare state as we know it – and it's often hard to find much common ground between these two opposing stances. Only half in jest has all this been dubbed a 'Marmite' issue – with personalisation rapidly emerging as something that people either love or hate.

Against this background, this edited collection brings together advocates and critics of personalisation in English social care services, including people with experience of using services, people working in services, people helping to reform services and people with experience of researching and teaching about the issues at stake. Whereas in the past people broadly favourable to and critical of personalisation have published separately, leading to accusations that they have side-lined or misrepresented alternative viewpoints, this book brings together a range of different voices and perspectives in one place. The advantage of such an approach is that it gives an overview of the diversity of opinion and experience that exists around the personalisation agenda – and reviewing the different contributions will hopefully enable readers (whether students, practitioners, managers, policymakers or academics) to reflect on the different stances taken, key areas of contention and possible areas of synergy. In the process, the differences of opinion expressed by different authors may also go a long way to explaining why personalisation is experienced in such different ways by different people in different parts of the country.

Of course, a downside of this approach is that someone new to the topic might find the different contributions a little disorientating at first reading. In one sense, there is not really any way round this – personalisation and its implementation is such a contentious issue that engaging with the various arguments at stake is almost inevitably disorientating. Almost by definition, different chapters are also written by people from different backgrounds, so the tone and approach is often different (ranging from reporting detailed research findings to very personal experiences and reflections). To do what we can to help, we have tried to make sure that all contributors write in a clear and accessible (if often challenging) style and that we present a range of different views so that readers can ultimately make up their own minds. We have also tried to reflect on our own in-built assumptions and beliefs in the process of editing the book, including one editor closely associated with In Control and widely seen as an advocate of direct payments and personalisation (see, for example, Glasby and Littlechild, 2009; Glasby et al, 2009; Duffy et al, 2010; Glasby, 2012a) and another with a track record for more critical and ambivalent analysis of personalisation and the way in which such terms are used in different ways by different stakeholders (see, for example, Needham, 2010a, 2011a, 2011b, 2013).

To provide as much structure as possible to these different views, the book is divided into five sections, focusing on:

- An introduction to/overview of the personalisation agenda (Chapters One to Three)
- Some of the key challenges of personalisation (Chapters Four to Eight)
- Frontline perspectives from service users, families, providers and staff (Chapters Nine to Twelve)
- The spread to healthcare (Chapters Thirteen to Sixteen)
- Overall responses to the issues raised (Chapters Seventeen to Nineteen)

We have not been able to cover in-depth all the issues associated with personalisation – for example we touch only briefly on the role of user-led organisations, and do not deal directly with reablement as part of personalised care services – but we hope to have included a diverse range of issues and perspectives that readers will find stimulating. The Care Act 2014 was also in the process of becoming law as the book was finalised, although the themes raised in the subsequent chapters remain pertinent despite the shifts in the precise legal context.

After this introduction, Chapter Two (by Catherine Needham and Jon Glasby) takes stock of the recent history of personalised social care services in England, reviewing the background of direct payments and person-centred approaches, considering how the *Putting People First* agenda is being implemented, highlighting the key controversies and considering the spread of personalisation to other areas of the welfare state. In Chapter Three, Sarah Carr summarises and critiques the broader policy context, with a particular focus on two key policies or initiatives (*Putting People First* and *Think Local, Act Personal*). Despite the rhetoric of personalisation becoming firmly established across government (and indeed surviving a change of government), tensions in broader policy can mean that implementation of such rhetoric into everyday practice can be challenging (to say the least).

In Chapter Four, Lucy Series focuses on the resource allocation systems (or RASs) that local authorities use to allocate indicative personal budgets – a crucial mechanism that was designed to allocate equal resources to equal levels of need but that can easily lead to significant problems (and indeed legal challenges) if not carefully designed and implemented. Particularly worrying is a lack of transparency over how such mechanisms work in practice (which feels ironic, given that the aim of personal budgets is to provide greater transparency and clarity of entitlement). After this, Chapter Five (by Jill Manthorpe) explores the relationship between personalisation and safeguarding. While these should be two sides of the same coin, they have often been seen as separate issues (particularly in the early days of personalisation), and further work has been needed to bring these two agendas closer together at both policy and practice level. In Chapter Six, Liz Lloyd asks if personalisation can work for older people, reviewing the common claim that personalised approaches as currently implemented may work better for people of working age. With older people making up the majority of social care users and in an ageing society, this is a serious charge, and one that cannot be resolved without exploring the broader social and cultural context of older people's services more generally.

In Chapter Seven, Wendy Mitchell, Jenni Brooks and Caroline Glendinning observe that carers have received relatively little attention to date in debates about personalisation, asking 'where do carers fit?' Presenting findings from the Carers and Personalisation study (2011- 13), they highlight difficulties for workers in overcoming separate legal frameworks and emphasise the importance of interdependence between 'users' and 'carers.' In Chapter Eight, Melanie Henwood explores the experience of self-funders – an often forgotten group of people who might be expected to have similar levels of choice and control over their support as envisaged by the personalisation agenda. In practice, this chapter argues that most self-funders do not find that their purchasing power necessarily leads to better outcomes, and there are more substantial barriers to greater independence in the current system than personal budgets alone might help to overcome.

Moving on to consider 'frontline perspectives' (Part Three), Christine Bond (Chapter Nine) reflects on her personal experiences of personal budgets and managing a direct payment. After some of the previous policy and research-based chapters, this is a very practical account of the benefits of personal budgets, some of the practical issues that need thinking through and what needs to be in place for personal budgets to work well. A crucial final line (p xx) acknowledges that 'this way of working is still bringing new challenges and everyone has to think differently for things to work well' – a succinct summary of many of the key issues perhaps. In Chapter Ten, Sian Lockwood describes the potential contribution of micro-enterprise to personalised care and support. Although many commentators acknowledge the need for new and innovative forms of service provision, it is still relatively rare to see such practical examples of provider innovation more widely debated. Describing her experience of working in this area as 'inspiring yet frustrating' (p xx), Sian illustrates the many barriers that can get in the way of new approaches and emphasises the hard work needed to make personalisation a reality.

In Chapter Eleven, UNISON's Helga Pile explores the neglect of workforce issues in many debates around personalisation. If we are not careful, the chapter warns, we could see a series of damaging changes to the social care workforce where both user and worker are ultimately disempowered. In Chapter Twelve, Victoria Hart offers a perspective as a frontline social worker, describing the commitment of many workers to more personalised approaches but also a strong sense that the personalisation agenda has 'over-promised and under-delivered' (p 112). Throughout there is an equal measure of passion about the potential of personalisation coupled with a deep sense of disillusionment and betrayal over the way in which policy has been implemented in practice.

Section Four moves on to consider the spread of personalisation from adult social care to the NHS, with a particular focus on personal health budgets. In Chapter Thirteen, Colin Royle talks movingly about his dad's dementia and about the way in which a personal health budget helped to restore the lives of the family as a whole. This is followed in Chapter Fourteen (by Julien Forder and Karen Jones) by more formal research findings from the national evaluation of personal health budgets. Despite a number of limitations, the study identifies some potential positives and provides support for the national roll-out of personal health budgets now taking place. In contrast, Chapter Fifteen (by Colin Slasberg) takes a different line, asking if personal health budgets pose a threat to the traditional values and ethos of the health service. If we are not careful, he argues, we could draw the wrong lessons from the evidence base, benefitting a small number of people at the expense of the majority and undermining the commitment of the NHS to notions of fairness and universalism. Vidhya Alakeson (Chapter Sixteen) reviews some of the challenges that personal health budgets entail, but also argues that this way of working can support greater self-management for people with long-term conditions and that we need to maintain the current political consensus around the importance of more personalised forms of healthcare.

Section Five then starts to explore a series of more cross-cutting themes, with Peter Beresford (Chapter Seventeen) and Simon Duffy (Chapter Eighteen) presenting potentially different versions of recent events and future possibilities. Both authors, in different ways, are key figures in the development of adult social care – and reading these two accounts side by side provides a series of fascinating insights into the issues at stake. Finally, Chapter Nineteen (by Jon Glasby and Catherine Needham) reflects on some of the key themes from the overall book, exploring the extent to which there are similarities and differences in the various contributions and asking whether there is scope for any degree of consensus in future. While some positive ways forward may be possible, it is difficult to avoid the impression that personalisation remains very much a 'Marmite issue' – deep down, readers will probably either love it or hate it.

TWO

Taking stock of personalisation

Catherine Needham and Jon Glasby

There has been growing interest in narrative approaches to policy that focus on how policies are framed as stories in order to build coalitions of support (Hajer, 1995; Yanow, 1996, 2000; Fischer, 2003). Such interpretive approaches to policy have also drawn attention to the ways in which academics themselves offer narrative interpretations of those policies: 'stories about stories' (Yanow, 1996). This layering of interpretation is very evident in relation to the recent changes to English social care services that are commonly referred to as personalisation. Personalisation has been variously described as a script, a rhetorical device and a set of stories that are told about care services and the people who use and work with them (Leadbeater, 2004; Needham, 2010b, 2011a; Ferguson, 2012). What is increasingly evident is that there are also lots of stories that academics and other stakeholders tell *about* personalisation: its genesis; its implementation; its impact; its future. These are not stories in the sense of being fictional or trivial. Rather they are competing narratives, which explain the past, present and future of personalisation in different ways.

The policy context

Perhaps the least contested element of personalisation is its policy locus. In a public policy context – as opposed to retail or technology where the term is also used – personalisation is usually applied to a set of policy changes to adult social care services in England from the mid-2000s. The term itself is commonly attributed to Charles Leadbeater in a 2004 Demos pamphlet in which he set out the key tenets of a personalised approach to public services, drawing on examples from social care (Leadbeater, 2004). The first major government policy statement on personalisation was the 2007 *Putting People First* concordat, signed by central government, local government and the social care sector (DH, 2007). This of course is not to claim that the policy sprang from thin air in the mid-2000s; its antecedents are highly contested, as discussed in the next section. However, a brief recent history can be sketched out with some confidence.

The 2007 *Putting People First* concordat set out the direction of adult social care reform over the next ten years. A 'transformation grant' of £520 million was made available to local authorities to promote personalisation, which incorporated the development of personal budgets, alongside more investment in prevention, better access to universal services and the development of social capital (DH, 2007). Reablement services were a key element of this agenda, aimed at fostering independence and keeping people out of statutory social care services for as long as possible (Francis et al, 2011). Councils were also required to set up a user-led organisation in each local authority and engage with service users and the wider community throughout the transformation process. However, it was personal budgets that were the highest profile strand of the personalisation reforms, becoming synonymous with personalisation for many commentators, despite reminders that the agenda was much broader than that (Fox, 2011a). National Indicator 130 required local authorities to have 30% of eligible service users on personal budgets by April 2011, affirming the message that budgets were the core priority within the personalisation agenda.

The personal budget target was extended to 100% of eligible users having a personal budget by 2013, generating concerns that pressures to increase the quantity of personal budgets were taking precedence over the quality of support being offered. As a result of such concerns, the target was revised down to 70% (Samuel, 2012). National bodies such as the Association of Directors of Adult Social Services (ADASS) and Think Local, Act Personal (TLAP), a partnership of social care bodies, were given a key role in supporting local authorities and care providers in making the transition to personalised approaches.

Many local authorities have put in place a resource allocation system (RAS) to calculate how much personal budget should be allocated to a user. Once a budget is allocated, people in receipt of social care funding should be able to choose to manage the money themselves as a direct payment or to have it managed by the local authority or a third party (as an individual service fund). A combination of these options should also be available. The person using services (along with their carer, where appropriate) and a support planner (who may be a social worker, another local authority employee, or a third party) then work to put together a support plan. Plans must be linked to approved outcomes and signed off by the local authority, but users are encouraged to be creative in how funds are spent – irrespective of whether the funds are held as a direct payment or a managed personal budget. Spending choices may be something very different from a traditional package of care services.

Survey figures from 2013 indicated that 76% of eligible people now hold a personal budget, although over two-thirds of these are managed personal budgets rather than direct payments (Samuel, 2013a). The Think Local, Act Personal team has expressed concern that people on managed personal budgets may not be seeing any substantive change in their support arrangements, with older people being a particular focus of concern (Routledge and Carr, 2013). The National Personal Budget survey in 2011 reported that 'older adults are less likely to use direct payments, less likely to know how their personal budget was managed, and more likely to have a personal budget managed by the council – all these factors are associated with less positive outcomes' (Hatton and Waters, 2011, p 26).

Personal budgets are now spreading from adult social care into other aspects of health and social care services. Pathfinder projects are under way for personal budgets for children with disabilities and with special educational needs (Teather, 2012). The Darzi reviews of the National Health Service (2007, 2008) proposed the piloting of personal health budgets (PHBs) within the NHS, drawing explicit inspiration from their perceived success in social care. These budgets are now being implemented nationally for those in receipt of Continuing Healthcare funding, with local areas also being encouraged to extend PHBs to people with long-term conditions (DH, 2012a; Forder, 2013).

The history

The formal policy changes in recent years are a matter of public record. However, once an account of personalisation strays beyond these formal boundaries, the contested nature of the concept becomes highly evident. The genesis of personalisation is one area of such controversy. Explaining its emergence as a policy issue in the mid-2000s involves giving an account of how two different policy streams intersected with the political agendas of the Conservative and New Labour governments of the 1980s and 1990s. These two streams were, first, the impetus for direct payments for people using social care services promoted by the independent living movement and centred on people with physical disabilities, and, second, the move to more inclusive approaches for people with learning disabilities.

Direct payments were a key element of campaigns for independent living from the 1980s, although explicitly prohibited under the founding legislation of the post-war welfare state. Such campaigns, and the willingness of some local authorities to work on the fringes of what was legally allowed, led to a more permissive environment towards cash payments to individuals, culminating in the Community Care (Direct Payments) Act 1996. The Act gave local authorities the power to make direct payments, which became a duty in 2001. Campaigners for direct payments drew on rights-based arguments but also on a cost-cutting rationale that was seen as more likely to attract support from John Major's Conservative government (Zarb and Nadash, 1994). As Glasby and Littlechild put it:

> While direct payments were a victory for disabled campaigners, they were also championed by a Conservative government committed to neo-liberal social policies aimed at rolling back the frontiers of the welfare state and promoting greater consumer choice through the creation of markets in social care. (2006, pp 27–8)

Direct payments were initially targeted towards people with physical disabilities. Within learning disability services, emphasis was increasingly being placed on inclusion and person-centred planning, in which control over financial resources was again seen as crucial to empowerment (O'Brien and Lyle O'Brien, 1998). Local authorities such as Wigan started experimenting with individualised budgets in learning disability services in the mid-2000s, drawing inspiration in part from the trialling of individual budgets that Simon Duffy had undertaken in Scotland (Duffy, 2010). Such budgets were more flexible than direct payments, based on the principle that people should have maximum choice and control over money spent on their behalf, including the freedom to spend it on anything that meets an assessed need (Glasby and Littlechild, 2009, p 76).

This experimentation caught the attention of national policymakers, partly through direct campaigning by disability rights groups and partly through the advocacy of the social innovation network In Control (which emerged out of the work being done in Wigan). Individual budgets for older people and people with disabilities were promoted in a series of government policy documents, culminating in *Putting People First* (DH, 2007). Difficulties in the implementation of individual budgets, which integrated funding from a range of sources, led to them being rechristened as personal budgets, and drawing only on social care funding.

The link between this experimentation and the ongoing practice of direct payments was often understated. Ministers and civil servants were keen to frame such budgets as a radical new approach to social care that cohered with their broader commitment to expanding user choice within public services. Clements notes the use of '"mould breaking" revolutionary language' in relation to individual budgets, despite an unchanged legal context for accessing care (2008, p 426). In Control supported this framing as part of a way of securing government support, while recognising that there was an element of 'the emperor's new clothes' about the agenda (Needham, 2011a). As Duffy observed, 'many long-standing practices are being re-described so that they are seen as part of the new zeitgeist' (2010, p 254). Beresford has been critical of the ahistorical ways in which he feels organisations such as Demos and In Control promoted the personalisation agenda: 'Individual budgets (IBs) and personal budgets (PBs) were advanced earlier in the noughties as a brave *new* idea. But the reality is they are precisely derived from the direct payments created and developed by the disabled people's movement almost a generation earlier' (2012, p 39).

Tensions between pragmatic accommodations to the government of the day and principled defences of the rights of people with disabilities (and 'top-down' versus 'bottom-up' accounts of change) are a recurrent theme within the history of personalisation. The hybrid rationale for the legalisation of direct payments in the 1990s – which harnessed government enthusiasm for cost-cutting and voucher-type approaches with disability rights campaigns – has become more pronounced as the policy has evolved into the more wide-ranging agenda of personalisation. Ferguson (2012, p 58) describes personalisation as the 'offspring of two discourses or ideologies [independent living and neo-liberalism] which, while both employing the language of independence, choice and control, have very different origins and aims'. He draws attention to four ways in which the independent living discourse differs from the neoliberal rationale:

> Its origins ('bottom-up', emerging out of collective movements rather than 'top-down'), its aims (social change and social justice, rather than simply involvement in services), ideology (a social, rather than an individual or biomedical model of health or disability) and its methods (often involving collective action, rather than 'partnership' with service providers). (Ferguson, 2008, p 70)

The 'powerful hybridisation' between market consumerism and social rights that was evident in the direct payments settlement has continued in the personalisation reforms (Scourfield, 2005, p 473). This hybridity can be interpreted as a strength of personalisation, enabling it to be endorsed by people across the political spectrum (Cutler et al, 2007). As Duffy puts it, personalisation is an 'appealing term that can be embraced by people with different political prejudices and preferences' (Duffy, 2010, p 255). However, Ferguson argues that this ambiguity has facilitated the silencing of progressive elements of the agenda:

> It is the 'market-consumer' or neoliberal discourse, now heavily underpinned by the austerity measures introduced by the current Coalition government in the UK, rather than the progressive agenda of the Disability Movement, which is currently the main ideological driver of personalisation. (2012, p 57)

There are parallels here with Stuart Hall's (2003) discussion of New Labour as a 'hybrid regime'. Considering the Blairite attempt to combine neoliberalism and social democracy, he argued:

> New Labour is a *hybrid* regime, composed of two strands. However, one strand – the neo-liberal – is in the dominant position. The other strand – the social democratic – is subordinate. What's more, its hybrid character is not simply a static formation; it is the *process* which combines the two elements which matters.... The latter always remains subordinate to and dependent on the former, and is *constantly being 'transformed'* into the former, dominant one. (2003, p 19, emphasis in original)

This account of hybridity as dynamic rather than static, and as a hierarchy rather than a process of mutual accommodation, resonates with many concerns about the development of personalisation.

The role of evidence

Another contested element of personalisation is the extent to which it has been based on formal evidence, or rather has proceeded on the basis of anecdotal claims about its effectiveness. Certainly, there is no shortage of formal evaluation data about personalisation. The Department of Health (DH) funded a major evaluation of individual budgets (Glendinning et al, 2008) and has subsequently funded a large-scale evaluation of personal health budgets (Forder et al, 2012). In Control runs a national evaluation each year, using the Personal Budgets Outcome and Evaluation Tool (POET). ADASS undertakes an annual survey on levels of take-up of personal budgets. Community Care and UNISON together have surveyed social work staff annually on their views of personalisation. Many other organisations have formally evaluated aspects of personalisation or undertaken evidence reviews to share best practice (for example, the Social Care Institute for Excellence, the Audit Commission, the Cabinet Office, and the New Local Government Network).

However, concerns have been expressed about the extent to which personalisation has been promoted on the basis of a shallow evidence base. As Beresford puts it: 'The narrative of individual/personal budgets was then sold powerfully through stories from some service users of new flexibility and opportunities in their lives, far better than reliance on traditional services' (2012, p 37). Individual testimonies have played a key role in establishing policy support for personalisation (Needham, 2011a). As a member of In Control put it, '"One of the things that we did very early on was start to tell positive stories about self directed support and how it was working, and that's what's captured the imagination"' (cited in Needham, 2011a).

It is possible to characterise diverse responses to the evidence base as the clash of different epistemological traditions – the formal and quantitative versus the qualitative and narrative-based – but that does not seem to be the key issue here. Rather, uneasiness about the evidence base comes from a sense that formal evidence is being used opportunistically and partially to substantiate a pre-determined policy position, affirming the importance of argument over evidence that has been a broader theme of critiques of 'evidence-based policy' (Sullivan, 2011).

Three aspects of the personalisation evidence base have drawn particular criticism.

Sequencing

The tendency of the implementation of personalisation to run ahead of the evidence base has been widely noted. As Beresford puts it:

> We then moved from a few pilot projects to a massive cash injection from central government to 'transform' social care and targets of moving service users to personal

budgets that ranged from one third to all....This was prior to the emergence of a strong body of evidence, when even before government had the results of its own research, it was committing itself to making massive policy change in favour of personal budgets. (2012, p 38)

A similar pattern was evident in the roll-out of the personal health budgets, with an announcement about national implementation for people on NHS Continuing Healthcare coming before the completion of the evaluation (DH, 2012a).

Interpretation

There are also controversies about how the data should be interpreted. Almost all the formal evaluation data has indicated that people who currently receive direct payments get better outcomes than those on managed personal budgets or traditional modes of funding, and there is little disagreement on this in the literature. However what this *means* is much more contested. The approach of the DH, TLAP and In Control has been to argue that the more people who receive direct payments, the more likely it is that better outcomes will be achieved. Making direct payments the default has become a priority of government social care policy.

Others have argued that there are characteristics of current direct payment holders that mean that it is invalid to generalise from their experience. Slasberg and colleagues (2012a, 2012b) have criticised the work of Hatton and others on the national POET survey, arguing that direct payment holders with relatively generous packages of support are overrepresented and are skewing the sample. Responding to similar criticisms in a *Community Care* debate with Slasberg, Hatton argued that further statistical testing of the survey data has refuted the claim that 'the positive impact of personal budgets is entirely a function of the increased resources received by holders of direct payments', finding that 'costs accounted for, at most, 7% of the variance in people's reports of impact' (Hatton and Slasberg, 2011). However, Slasberg and colleagues express continued dissatisfaction with the lack of transparency over the statistical tests used (2012b, p 1033).

Slasberg has also argued that current direct payment holders are more likely than the broader population of people with disabilities to have networks of support, enabling them to access the benefits that such payments can bring (Hatton and Slasberg, 2011). He argues that:

> People with direct payments tend to be highly articulate people able to negotiate their way through powerful interests, including council officers. It is likely that this personal powerfulness not only accounts for their enthusiasm to act as their own commissioner, but also explains why they have higher funding than most. (Hatton and Slasberg, 2011)

Hatton's rejoiner to Slasberg in the *Community Care* debate highlights the intensity of the debate about interpretation of the data:

> It puzzles me why his hostility is directed towards personal budgets, when his concerns (which I share) about inequality, lack of transparency and accountability, bureaucracy and unresponsive services have been pervasive concerns about traditional social services cultures and practices long before personal budgets came on the scene. (Hatton and Slasberg, 2012)

What is the relevant evidence?

A further point of contention has been what sort of evidence is relevant in assessing the impact of personalisation. Much of the data has quite rightly focused on the experience of people using services, as discussed above. However, some people have argued that the user experience needs to be supplemented with other forms of evidence to give a truer picture of whether or not personalisation is fulfilling its aims. A number of authors have focused attention on resource allocation systems (RASs), points-based systems that local authorities use to provide an 'up-front allocation' (Fox, 2011b; Slasberg et al, 2012a; Series and Clements, 2013). This allocation is a key part of the personal budget process as established by In Control's Seven Steps to Self-Directed Support, marking a distinction from traditional approaches to allocation in which funding allocations occur after appropriate support is identified and are often invisible to the person receiving support.

The DH has recognised that the RAS may produce a figure that needs to be adjusted in order to ensure that eligible needs can be met, but TLAP has made clear that 'the indicative allocation amount should be as close as possible to the final approved budget' (TLAP, 2011, p 8). However, Series and Clements (2013) and Slasberg and colleagues (2012a) find evidence that there is so little match between the RAS allocation and the final budget as to throw into doubt the validity of the RAS process. Looking at figures from a series of local authorities, Slasberg and colleagues conclude that 'the "sign off" of the budget appears to be not so much a quick check on whether the figure created by the up-front allocation is enough but an entirely separate decision that stands alone from the up-front process' (2012a, p 164). Similarly, having reviewed 20 RASs, following a Freedom of Information request, Series and Clements conclude: 'The RAS appears to be a cog spinning inside a machine with which it does not engage. It neither reduces the labour of social care assessment, nor provides service users with enforceable "entitlements"' (2013, p 225). Slasberg and colleagues conclude that 'there is a serious question as to whether personal budgets, as they are defined, exist at all' (2012a, p 170).

A second set of data has focused on the impact on social care staff, for example in terms of additional bureaucracy. A UNISON/*Community Care* poll of social care staff from 2010 showed that two-thirds of respondents had experienced increased bureaucracy as a result of personalisation. This figure had risen to 82% by 2012 (Donovan, 2012). A number of studies (for example, Jacobs et al, 2011; Slasberg et al, 2012a) have found that assessments for personal budgets are taking longer than traditional assessments, leaving less time for reviews of service packages for existing users. This appears to be due in part to local authorities duplicating self-assessments and traditional community care assessments, because of a fear that legal duties to assess people's needs would not otherwise be met (Samuel, 2010). Frustration at such practices, which distort the transparency and simplicity that advocates of personal budgets envisaged, has come from many quarters (for example, Jerome, 2010; Routledge, 2011; Duffy, 2012a).

What has personalisation achieved?

Those who have been supportive of personalisation and those who have been critical of it agree that the key criterion against which personalisation should be judged is that of social justice (Duffy, 2010; Ferguson, 2012). Yet of course this is a difficult measure to use with any element of standardisation. There is also disagreement about how far personalisation should be modified or abandoned because of inadequacies in relation to social justice that are external to personalisation (such as the underfunding of social care, and society's perception and treatment of older people and people with disabilities).

There is recognition by many people writing on personalisation that it has not achieved what it set out to achieve. According to Beresford (2012, p 40):

From a means to empowerment, we have moved to what is essentially an under-funded voucher system. From a replacement for a traditional and inadequate set of services, we have moved to an exchange relationship, which casts the service user as a consumer, not a citizen with rights – to a model that is market based and market driven rather than liberatory in intent.

Duffy, one of the most active proponents of self-directed support, has acknowledged that the achievements of personalisation have been limited: 'the reality is that personalisation, with all the hope it offers, is never going to deliver either a decent or a fair society – unless we put in place a constitutional framework to protect the rights and entitlements of disabled people' (2012a, p 24).

There are a range of views about why personalisation has thus far failed to achieve its goals. For some authors, as discussed earlier in the chapter, personalisation is a 'Trojan horse' for neoliberalism, advancing a policy agenda designed to reduce state welfare services and deprofessionalise workers (see, for example, Ferguson, 2007, 2012; Lloyd, 2010; Barnes, 2011; Roulstone and Prideaux, 2012). An alternative interpretation is that personalisation is a well-meaning policy that has been derailed – either by the massive funding cuts that have been imposed since 2010 – or by local forms of implementation that have sought to reinvent traditional approaches under a personalisation heading (as in the complex and ineffective RASs) (Routledge, 2010; Duffy, 2012a). Concerns about bureaucracy and legal ambiguity have been highlighted earlier in this chapter. A third explanation is that the gap between the promise and the reality of personalisation is a temporal one: personalisation has not yet had time to establish itself as a mainstream approach to adult social care services, although the benefits of extending direct payments have been established. The key response then is to keep faith with personalisation and ensure that it does not suffer the fate of earlier reforms. As former personalisation lead at the DH Martin Routledge puts it, 'I was there in 1993 when care management came in. We simply must make sure that doesn't happen again' (Routledge, 2010). Beresford (2012, p 37), however, includes personalisation as one of the failed innovations of social care:

Social care's history is littered with previous examples of such overclaimed and inadequately evidenced innovations, from 'patch' social services in the 1980s through to care

management in the 1990s. All of these have subsequently
been seen to fail.

These contending explanations together contribute to an understanding
of why the achievements of personalisation to date have been limited.
Ideology, timescales, financing and local interpretation all sustain the
complex link between a policy initiative and changes in frontline
practice. The ambiguity and indeterminacy of the policy, discussed
earlier, is crucial here, and (along with funding cuts) may play a
bigger role in explaining partial implementation than deliberate
subversion by managers or frontline staff, or a coherent, omnipotent,
neoliberal ideology. The disconnect between the promise and reality
of personalisation reflects social care policies in which managers and
staff are expected to achieve multiple, cross-cutting if not directly
contradictory goals, such as more tailored services, at the same time
as massive funding cuts (Needham, 2013). In discussing how best to
understand such an 'implementation gap', Ball (1997, p 265) argues:
'When ensembles of uncoordinated or contradictory policies are in play
then the resort to satisficing strategies and secondary accommodations
may be the only reasonable and feasible response in certain points in
time'. In other words, apparent delivery failures may be indicative of the
pressures facing frontline social care services, which limit the scope for
meaningful implementation at a time of an urgent short-term funding
crisis and a long-term funding shortfall.

Where should personalisation go next?

One of the features of personalisation is that it has spun out from
adult social care into a range of other policy domains. The language of
personalised services is now used in a range of sectors from employment
to prisons to school building design and the education curriculum. The
technologies of personal budgets are being utilised widely, including
children's social care, special educational needs provision, rough sleepers
and NHS services. The most wide-ranging of these is the personal
health budgets programme, which constitutes a radical change to NHS
funding for people with long-term conditions.

What should be read into this policy migration is disputed. Partly it
reflects the breadth of ambition of some of those, such as Duffy, who
sought to promote personalised approaches to social care. The principles
of entitlement, set out by Duffy and others, are not easily bound by a
policy sector, and he is keen to see self-directed approaches expanded
into a range of sectors such as education, with a corresponding change

to the tax and benefits system (Duffy et al, 2010; Duffy, 2011a). It is also, arguably, a reflection of the desire of government for grand policy narratives, which can lend a sense of coherence to reforms across public services.

However two key issues are raised when considering the expansion of personalisation and personal budgets across public services. The first is how far the evidence base in social care is robust enough to support this expansion. Disputes over what can be inferred from the evidence are set out earlier in the chapter. The implementation of personalisation in adult social care services has been patchy and its impact on outcomes is contestable. It remains unclear whether it is an agenda that will reshape the entire market of care services, driving up choice and quality, or will make a difference to a few thousand direct payment holders who can realise its promise of more choice and control. Both of these constitute important changes to care services, which have often failed to deliver quality or dignity to the people using them, but they have very different implications at a system level. There is also an obvious concern over how far quality and dignity can be achieved without adequate funding and worries that government proposals on changes to the funding of social care will not bring sufficient money into the system.

The second issue is how far the distinctive features of social care services make extensions into other service areas problematic. A very different funding model operates in health, based on universal provision rather than means-testing. The NHS was established on the basis that rationing would be largely invisible to the patient, and that risk would be pooled across the community of taxpayers and non-taxpayers. The disaggregation of health spending into personal health budgets has been seen by some as a major challenge to that payment system and the collective principles on which it is based. Certainly, there has been a disconnect between the promotion of personal budgets in social care and initiatives to encourage more collaborative working between health and social care services (for example in relation to hospital discharge) (Glendinning et al, 2011).

Education is traditionally provided in a collective school setting, unlike the more individualised service models that dominate in health and social care. If education were to be provided on the basis of parents choosing to opt in to different bits of provision, using a voucher or other form of disaggregated budget, there would be clear concerns about this facilitating segregation and inequality. However, children with profound learning disabilities and/or physical impairments might already be accessing education and health/social care services that embody these tensions – and a broader approach based around greater self-directed support could be a way of accommodating such dilemmas. Thus, each service area will raise a distinctive set of issues – about the delivery of the service, the user–professional relationship and the framing of 'expertise' – which means that personalisation needs to be considered afresh in that context.

Conclusion

This chapter has highlighted the ambiguity of personalisation as an approach to policy and the indeterminacy of its evidence base. Ferguson's point is an important one:

> [T]here is no 'true' meaning of personalisation any more than there is a 'true' meaning of empowerment or participation or choice. Rather, these are contested concepts, terrains of political struggle and debate on which different social forces seek to impose their preferred meaning. (Ferguson, 2012, p 57)

However, this is no more true of personalisation than it is of a wide range of concepts in social science (Gallie, 1955). The aim of this chapter (and the book as a whole) is not to abandon readers in a fog of ambivalence. The chapters that follow present a range of perspectives and data on how personalisation is developing, which provide insight into different elements of the agenda. However, it is hoped that they will also remind readers that policies are developed on the basis of argumentation, ideology and emotion as well as formal evidence. Scholars of public policy, people using services and frontline practitioners all bring their own interpretive lenses, informed by ideologies and epistemologies that may be inexplicit and incommensurable. Attitudes to risk and expectations of the state are essentially contested and yet are crucial to the deployment of social care policies. Points of common agreement – the chronic underfunding of care services, the importance of maintaining dignity and control for people using services – lead authors to very different conclusions.

THREE

Making it real: from *Putting People First* to *Think Local, Act Personal*

Sarah Carr

This chapter is a critical examination of the core government personalisation policy documents – *Putting People First* (DH, 2007) and *Think Local, Act Personal* (TLAP, 2011b) – and how the proposals were influenced by broader strategies for welfare reform. It analyses the policy documents across changing ideological standpoints following the 2010 change of government from New Labour to a Conservative-dominated coalition with the Liberal Democrats. The intention is not to assess the implementation of all the personalisation policy reforms set out in the key government documents, but rather to examine the documents as artefacts of the broader welfare and public policy reform ideologies of the different administrations. In this way it is possible to explore how some of the wider government public sector reform strategies have shaped personalisation implementation proposals. The methodology is informed by a documentary analysis approach. This exploration of key personalisation policy documents highlights how they bear the hallmarks of wider welfare reform approaches in both administrations and draws on critical perspectives offered by selected academics. The analysis draws on research-based explorations of the 'modernisation' and 'transformation' reform agendas in adult social care (Newman et al, 2008), refers to a critique of joined-up government (Pollitt, 2003) and traces adult social care policy evolution (Means, 2012). Evidence is drawn from findings from the individual budgets (IB) pilot evaluation (Glendinning et al, 2011; Moran et al, 2011).

Policy evolution

Means (2012) offers a helpful historical perspective for contexualising personalisation reforms in adult social care. He sees the agenda as belonging within a historical continuum of policy development, where major themes about funding, quality, provision, access and defining social care continually re-emerge as challenges. Means argues that 'it needs to be remembered that the Griffiths Report is now over 20 years old and in many ways it set out the personalisation agenda which the coalition government now intends to implement' (2012, p 317). The 2007 *Putting People First* policy concordat refers back to the Community Care reforms instigated by Griffiths and the initial coalition adult social care reform document refers to the 1968 Seebohm Report, again highlighting the evolutionary nature of the policy. In their extensive examination of the New Labour social care and welfare 'modernisation' reform programme, from which the personalisation agenda emerged, Newman and colleagues (2008, p 532) recognise the evolutionary nature of modernisation in adult social care:

> Despite the charge that modernisation has not been a coherent programme of reform, it is nevertheless possible to trace its evolution within social care from the 1998 White Paper *Modernising social services* (DH, 1998) to *Independence, wellbeing and choice* (DH, 2005) and *Our health, our care, our say* (DH, 2006).

Their argument that New Labour health and social care modernisation had 'multiple trajectories of reform' could also be applied to personalisation, which became a core means for 'transformation' (Spicker, 2012). Newman and colleagues outline the argument that the policy shift from the systemic 'transactional' to the 'transformational' involves changing 'values, attitudes and relationships' and has the 'capacity to generate commitment rather than compliance [and] assume that a strong value base is of critical importance' (Newman et al, 2008 p 539). It is this type of value-based working and commitment that is presented in the *Putting People First* agreement of December 2007, which first introduced a policy narrative and implementation proposals for personalisation in adult social care. Indeed, the document is sub-headed 'A shared vision and commitment to the transformation of adult social care' (DH, 2007).

Putting People First

It has been argued that *Putting People First* articulated a reform programme for personalisation based on pre-existing modernisation policy proposals for health, social care and disability (Newman et al, 2008; Boxall et al, 2009). The document was presented as a concordat between multiple government departments, the NHS and numerous social care stakeholder organisations. It is important to note the collaborative intention for policy implementation, which reflects the scope and ambition of the associated personalisation reforms. The policy is published by HM Government, rather than a single ministerial department such as the Department of Health. As such the document and proposals also reflect a defining trope of New Labour public sector reform – 'joined-up government' (Pollitt, 2003). Reflecting Means' (2012) perspectives on policy evolution, the *Putting People First* document acknowledges that 'while … the Community Care legislation of the 1990s was well intentioned, it has led to a system which can be over complex and too often fails to respond to people's needs and expectations' (DH, 2007, p 1). In order to avoid associating the choice and flexibility offered by personalisation with the shortcomings of care management in the 1990s, the *Putting People First* approach is presented as transformational rather than transactional. As anticipated by Newman and colleagues (2008) in their analysis of transformational change in adult social care modernisation, *Putting People First* emphasises that personalisation is based on shared values and should be achieved through systemic collaboration across the public sector but without recourse to structural changes. Commentators have noted the 'common sense rationale' and the 'claim to self-evidence' of the personalisation values and principles presented in *Putting People First* (Needham, 2011b, p 57, 60). Among other delivery strategy proposals, the concordat document states that the Department of Health would lead a 'new cross-ministerial group … to ensure a joined-up approach to adult social care transformation' to drive the required changes from the centre (DH, 2007, p 4).

Joined-up government and individual budgets

To assess the extent to which the intended collaboration between *Putting People First* signatories, including the NHS, was realised, it is helpful to examine some of the less well-known findings from the IB pilot evaluation (Glendinning et al, 2008). As discussed elsewhere in this book, IBs represented an attempt by government to merge different funding streams and rationalise administrative processes in order to improve efficiency and increase choice and control for the individual. As such, they are a classic example of intended 'joined-up government', described by Pollitt (2003) as a strategy aimed at increasing policy effectiveness and reducing policy tensions or contradictions. However, in reality, this ambitious joined-up governmental reform became an example of fragmentation and duplication. IBs were initially introduced as a concept by the Prime Minister's Strategy Unit as part of the 2005 improving the life chances of disabled people policy proposals, of which the Department of Health, the Department for Work and Pensions and the Department for Education and Skills were signatories (PMSU, 2005). Notably, the proposed IBs did not include any NHS money (Henwood and Hudson, 2007) but the life chances proposals included investment in the infrastructure of user-led Centres for Independent Living (later known in policy as User Led Organisations) to support IB implementation. Despite their origins in disability policy, IBs eventually became known as an approach to achieving personalised adult social care and leadership came to rest with the Department of Health. Nonetheless, ministerial departments, such as the Department for Work and Pensions and the Department for Communities and Local Government, were *Putting People First* signatories and responsible for several of the IB funding streams. Associated proposals for local authorities to support at least one User Led Organisation also appeared in the reform policies presented in *Putting People First*. However, the responsibility for their development lay with the Office for Disability Issues at the Department for Work and Pensions as part of the separate cross-government independent living strategy (ODI, 2008). In their evaluation of the Department of Health self-directed support network that supported the IB pilots and preceded *Putting People First*, Henwood and Hudson concluded that 'central government needs to address the remaining complexities that cannot be resolved locally and necessitate clarification ... and legislative resolution' (Henwood and Hudson, 2007 p 10).

Moran and colleagues (2011) argue that in practice it proved difficult, if not impossible, to integrate the different support funding sources at a local level. Further to this, Glendinning and colleagues (2011) report the consequences of excluding NHS funding from IBs for local health and social care collaboration. These findings provide examples of the tensions and complications for achieving the top-level collaboration set out in *Putting People First*. Moran and colleagues (2011) assert that 'despite the promotion of IBs as an example of joined-up government, tensions remained, often related to legal constraints on the use and accountability of different funding streams' (p 234). Based on the reports of lead officers in the IB pilot sites, they go on to argue that 'national legislation effectively prohibited integration at local level' (Moran et al, 2011, p 239). It is notable that *Putting People First* was published before the IB pilot evaluation was reported (Beresford, 2009), and introduced personal budgets only consisting of social care funding, yet it was presented as a 'joined-up government' policy. Moran and colleagues emphasise that by the time *Putting People First* appeared, 'attempts to include other funding streams appeared to have been abandoned' and yet 'the active engagement of [*Putting People First* ministerial signatories] would have arguably assisted considerably in enabling the IB pilot projects to make greater progress in integrating funding streams' (Moran et al, 2011, p 239). The Department for Work and Pensions and the Department for Communities and Local Government funding streams that could not be integrated were subsequently subject to the 'Right to Control Trailblazer' evaluation, led by the Office for Disability Issues (Tu et al, 2013). As explored in Chapter Sixteen in this book, personal health budgets were also subject to separate testing for the NHS (Forder et al, 2012). Moran and colleagues argue that these developments along with the lack of success in integrating funding streams and processes in IBs 'exemplify a profound failure of joined-up government. Indeed, rather than moving towards greater flexibility and integration of resource streams, the subsequent proliferation of individual-budget type initiatives carries the imprint of individual departmental resource and ministerial silos' (Moran et al, 2011, p 240).

Glendinning and colleagues (2011) also draw on the IB pilot findings to demonstrate the effects of the explicit exclusion of NHS resources from IBs, which they say 'appeared inconsistent with the previous decade of policies that had encouraged collaboration between health and social care' (2011, p 153). Analysis of interviews with local lead officers suggests 'how the contexts of local collaboration [between health and social care] created problems for the implementation of the personalisation pilots, jeopardised inter-sectorial relationships and threatened some of the collaborative arrangements that had developed over the previous decade', particularly for mental health (Glendinning et al, 2011, p151).

Again, this outcome appears at odds with the transformative ambitions for personalisation as outlined in *Putting People First*, which makes it clear that partnerships and collaboration with the NHS are key elements of a transformed, personalised adult social care system. It reflects Newman and colleagues' (2008) observation that modernisation reform has been characterised by multiple and sometimes incompatible pressures.

Think Local, Act Personal

The term 'personalisation' and much associated policy language transferred into the adult social care reform agenda of the coalition government from 2010. This included a similar exhortation to overarching, self-evident shared values (or what Newman and colleagues [2008] call 'super-ordinate goals') of independence, control, wellbeing and choice. As Boxall and colleagues (2009, p 508) have commented, 'because it is difficult to argue against personal choice and control, there is therefore an in-built bias towards – rather than away from – policy change that supports personalisation'. However, the style of government was different; it was not characterised by centrally driven joined-up government but by radical devolution of decision making and responsibility to local actors. The ideological discourse of the new administration appeared throughout the policy document *A vision for adult social care*, with an emphasis on individual responsibility, 'dependency' reduction and increasing community capacity. The underpinning rationale is that 'if power and control is devolved to communities, then people – including the most vulnerable – can lead more independent and fulfilled lives' (DH, 2010a, p 7). The proposal for the continued implementation of personalisation was not through a national and regional infrastructure, with the Department of Health taking a leadership role by hosting a central government support team. Instead, key players were asked to determine the direction and progress of the reforms:

> Reform cannot and will not be top-down. We want decision-making devolved as closely to the individual as possible, and we need the care services sector, working with partners, to take a lead role in promoting and delivering transformation. The Partnership Agreement *Think Local, Act Personal*, developed together with partners in the adult social care sector, set out concrete steps to transform social care. (DH, 2010a, p 7)

The discourse of personalisation remained intact in the preliminary coalition adult social care policy reform document, but the proposed implementation strategy was different and reflects the administration's broader welfare and public policy reforms around 'smaller government', devolution and localism. Further to this, the emphasis on 'capable communities' and volunteering was explicitly linked to the Conservatives' flagship 'Big Society' social policy idea (Cameron, 2009, p 9): 'We need a Big Society approach to social care – one that gives people the power to support each other and meet the challenges they face'. While *Putting People First* included reference to social care policy ancestry by critiquing the outcomes of the 1990 Community Care reforms, *A vision for adult social care* opened with reference to words from the 1968 Seebohm Report as the foundational touchstone for the reforms:

> Frederick Seebohm ... said that social care should enable 'the greatest possible number of individuals to act reciprocally, giving and receiving service for the well-being of the whole community'. We need a return to these foundations. (DH, 2010a, p 5)

While they remain part of the overall personalisation strategy, personal budgets and self-directed support appear alongside increased references to the amorphous concept of 'community' as the central means for implementing personalisation: 'personalisation can also be achieved by harnessing the untapped potential of communities'(DH, 2010a, p 17).

With the emphatic promotion of community-based support as integral to personalisation, the *Think Local, Act Personal* (TLAP) agreement is an example of the devolved approach to policy implementation. Although the strategy is presented as a collaboration, the signatories are not multiple central government departments. Rather, it is the Department of Health alone that sits alongside over 30 adult social care sector organisations, charities and provider agencies who volunteered to endorse the approach. The agreement is explicit about continuity with *Putting People First* but a different approach to implementation is proposed in line with the broader reform ideologies in *A vision for adult social care*. Instead of being accompanied by a local authority circular containing directive plans for change, the TLAP agreement itself forms the 'general framework for action' to be 'supported by examples to assist partners in benchmarking progress, and by co-designed tools to aid delivery' (TLAP, 2011b). The latter part of this proposal bears the hallmark of one of the ways in which decentralisation was initially instrumentalised by the coalition government – the scrapping of National Performance Indicators (such as NI130 designed to increase the uptake of personal budgets [DH, 2008; NAO, 2011]) and data returns (addressed in the 2010 'zero-based review' [DH, 2010g]) in preference for loose frameworks and optional guidelines. This wider development was most clearly articulated for adult social care in the introduction to the adult social care outcomes framework (ASCOF), which corresponded with the continued personalisation agenda:

> The Government will not seek to performance manage councils in relation to any of the measures set out in this framework. Instead, the ASCOF will inform and support

improvement led by the sector itself, underpinned by strengthened transparency and local accountability. (DH, 2012b, p 5)

Further, the responsible ministers emphasised that 'councils have been given the freedom to set and act on their own priorities, driven by the needs of local people, not of Whitehall' (DH, 2012b, p 3). Newman and colleagues argue that even as part of New Labour reforms, personal budgets indicated that 'government ... is now turning away from "top-down" levers that focus on structures and systems towards a reliance on service users themselves ... to lever change through the ways in which they exercise choice' (Newman et al, 2008, p 548).

One of the tasks of the TLAP partnership was to produce some 'markers of progress'. These were produced with people who use services and carers to provide a tool to aid implementation; a framework for reflection on performance; and to promote the status of people who use support and carers, changing them from consumers to citizens and community actors (a tension consistently present in personalisation, as explored throughout this book). In the resulting document, named *Making it real*, the progress markers are constituted as 'I statements', focusing the reader on the person who is on the receiving end and offering the individual a set of expectations with which to hold providers to account. The document further elucidates the character of the new phase for implementing personalisation: 'We use a citizen-focused agenda to change the kind of information that the sector values, and the way in which we judge success' (TLAP, 2011c, p 2). Instead of being expected to meet data-driven central performance targets, councils are encouraged to sign up to the initiative on a voluntary basis and 'take responsibility for change and publicly share progress being made' (TLAP, 2011c, p 2). At the time of writing, it is too early to assess how well this devolved and voluntary approach to embedding personalisation, with an emphasis on developing 'capable communities', is working. However, in the context of financial austerity and large cuts to public sector spending that have negative consequences for individual personal budget holders, carers and communities, it is evident that there are extreme policy contradictions (Wood and Grant, 2010; Carr, 2012; Lymbery, 2012).

Conclusion

The questions raised here through the work of Newman and colleagues (2008) and Means (2012) about the deeper issues of welfare governance, tensions, contradictions and continuums in adult social care policy help an analysis of personalisation's fundamental policy documents, *Putting People First* (DH, 2007), *Think Local, Act Personal* (TLAP, 2011b) and *Making it Real* (TLAP, 2011c). One aspect of implementation, IBs, demonstrates the challenges and complexities of achieving change through top-level 'joined-up government' and demonstrates that the ambitions set out in the policy document were far harder to achieve in reality. The exploration here shows that the rhetoric of personalisation has survived a change in government. This supports the view that 'the current emphasis on personalisation, independence and choice in adult social care is now firmly embedded across government discourse, organisational missions and professional norms of good practice. Yet ... these are unevenly inscribed in organisational and professional practice' (Newman et al, 2008, p 546). As this chapter has shown, despite the survival of personalisation as a policy narrative, its implementation is influenced by larger and sometimes contradictory welfare reforms, whatever the character of the government. This character forms a watermark in reform policy documents such as *Putting People First* and *Think Local, Act Personal*.

Part Two
The challenges of personalisation

FOUR

Resource allocation systems: complex and counterproductive?

Lucy Series

Background: the aims of resource allocation systems

Resource allocations systems (RASs) are computer algorithms used by local authorities to produce an 'indicative amount' for a personal budget, which service users and care practitioners may use to start planning their support. Most RASs work by allocating a point score to a person's responses on a needs questionnaire, and then converting that – using some algorithm – to a cash value. Some simplified RASs, called 'ready reckoners', require local authority staff to estimate how many hours of support per week they believe a person would need, and multiply this by an assumed unit cost of that care to arrive at a cash value.

It was hoped, when RASs were developed, that they would lead to a more fair, transparent and equitable distribution of resources in social care: more fair, because it was hoped that these algorithms would be less subjective than individual professional judgement (Duffy, 2005a); more transparent because they would make visible 'decision making processes that would otherwise be hidden' (Henwood and Hudson, 2007, p iii; see also Tyson, 2009; ADASS, 2010); and more equitable because they would eliminate institutionalised inequalities between different client groups with equivalent needs (Henwood and Hudson, 2007; EHRC, 2010).

By providing service users with a personal budget, rather than a care plan devised by professionals, it was hoped that service users would be 'empowered' to take control of their own care and support. By reducing the emphasis on professional assessment, and offering service users greater opportunities to plan their own care, it was envisaged that they would also reduce bureaucracy in adult social care. These are all laudable goals, yet growing evidence suggests that RASs are not operating in any of the ways anticipated by those who promoted them. This can, in part, be understood by looking at the discrepancy between what the law requires of local authority care service provision and how RASs work in practice. This chapter first considers the law, and then looks at empirical evidence about how RASs operate.

The legal status of RASs

As Clements (2008) has noted, RASs are creatures of policy not law; they are not referenced in any existing community care legislation. The government actively chose *not* to place RASs on any statutory footing in the Care Act 2014, which replaces and consolidates existing community care laws (DH, 2013a). Despite the government encouraging the use of RASs (DH, 2008, para 19; 2010c, paras 129, 130, 132), authorities are under no legal obligation to adopt a RAS system.

The law surrounding local authority assessment of need and provision of community care services remains largely untouched, despite the introduction of 'personalisation' policies. Authorities must assess a person's community care needs if it appears to them that the person may be eligible for services that they could provide (National Health Service and Community Care Act 1990, s 47). This assessment must comply with binding guidance (DH, 2010c), and qualifying carers must be offered a carers' assessment (Carers (Recognition and Services) Act 1995; Carers and Disabled Children Act 2000). Authorities must identify any needs that are 'eligible' for services, according to the eligibility threshold adopted in their area, and any eligible needs *must* be met, *regardless* of the cost of meeting those needs (*R v Gloucestershire County Council & Anor ex parte Barry* [1997] UKHL 58). Authorities may provide community care services to meet assessed eligible needs under an array of statutes (for example, the National Assistance Act 1948, the Chronically Sick and Disabled Persons Act 1970, and Mental Health Act 1983, s 117).

People who are eligible for community care services may request a 'direct payment' in lieu of services to spend on meeting their eligible needs, and provided certain conditions are met authorities are obliged to comply (Community Care (Direct Payments) Act 1996; Health and Social Care Act 2001; Health and Social Care Act 2008). Neither statute, regulations nor binding guidance prescribes how the value of a direct payment should be determined, but authorities making direct payments are still under the same legal obligation to ensure that a person's eligible needs for community care services are met. They are also under an obligation to have regard to economy, efficiency and effectiveness in discharging these duties (Local Government Act 1999). Authorities may levy charges against a 'personal budget' (DH, 2010b). As public authorities in the meaning of s6 Human Rights Act 1998, authorities must discharge their duties to provide care services in a way that is compatible with the person's human rights. This patchwork of disparate community care statutes has now been consolidated in the Care Act 2014.

A series of court cases has considered how the use of RASs fits in with this picture. In public law, if a public authority adheres rigidly to a blanket policy on how it exercises a discretionary power or duty, this is known as 'fettering its discretion', and forms grounds for a judicial review of decisions made under that policy. Public authorities can adopt policies prescribing how they discharge their powers and duties, but they must retain a residual discretion to depart from them should the circumstances require it. RASs risk 'fettering' a local authority's discretion in how they discharge their community care obligations to meet eligible needs, if they do not increase (or decrease) the value of a personal budget above the indicative amount produced by the RAS where necessary. In *R (JL) v Islington LBC* [2009] EWHC 458 (Admin), the High Court held that a local authority had acted unlawfully by failing to retain any residual discretion to increase an allocation by a points-based RAS where it was necessary (para 108). Although in many cases the hours awarded by the system would be sufficient, there could be no certainty that the system would, in every case, be sufficient to meet the needs of the particular person (para 106). Guidance on the Care Act 2014 states that personal budgets devised by a RAS must be 'sufficient' and 'one size fits all' approaches must be avoided (DH, 2014, paras 11.22-11.23).

One of the dangers with RASs is that by converting an entitlement to have eligible needs met to a cash entitlement, it may not be clear – either to the local authority or the service user – whether their needs *can* in fact be met within this financial envelope. Two cases have considered this issue. In *R (Savva) v Royal Borough of Kensington and Chelsea* [2010] EWCA Civ 1209, the Court of Appeal considered whether the local authority was obliged to give reasons for its decision to allocate Mrs Savva the same sum of money despite an increase in her needs. The court noted that neither statute nor regulations imposed a duty to give reasons (para 19); however, it found that a duty to give reasons arose out of a common law requirement for *fairness*:

> When a local authority converts an established right – the provision of services to meet an assessed eligible need – into a sum of money, the recipient is entitled to be told how the sum has been calculated.... If a local authority were entitled to notify a bald figure without any explanation,

the recipient would have no means of satisfying himself or herself that it was properly calculated. As the guidance from the Association of Directors of Social Services puts it, explanations of decisions 'make it possible for people and families to challenge these decisions'. Or, to put it the other way round, an absence of explanations may make it impossible to mount such a challenge, whether by way of complaint or by way of litigation. (para 20)

The Court of Appeal felt that the reasons could be given with reasonable brevity in most cases; it would be adequate to list the required services and assumed timings with the assumed hourly cost, although more expansive reasoning might be needed in more complex cases. The court also said that people had a right to know about the RAS itself, but that this could be achieved – as ADASS (2010) has recommended – by 'publishing the RAS on the Council's website in a user-friendly format' (para 21).

This reasoning was endorsed by the Supreme Court in *R (KM) v Cambridgeshire County Council* [2012] UKSC 23, where Lord Wilson agreed that there was a danger that when a person is allocated a global sum of money, 'a local authority's failure to meet eligible needs may prove to be far less visible' (para 36). Lord Wilson endorsed the approach given in *Savva*, of checking that a person's eligible needs could be met within the financial envelope, by listing the required services and assumed timings with the assumed cost (para 37). Although the Supreme Court agreed that it might be rational to use a RAS, this was only where the result was cross-checked to ensure it was adequate to meet assessed eligible needs.

In summary, the use of RASs has not been found to be unlawful. However, authorities' underlying obligation to meet assessed eligible needs must be discharged in full – even if that means *increasing* the value of a personal budget that was calculated by a RAS. It is the responsibility of the local authority to reassure itself that the value of the personal budget is capable of meeting assessed eligible needs, and it may do this by providing some kind of support plan with costings. It must supply its reasoning that the value of the personal budget is sufficient to meet their assessed eligible needs to service users or their supporters, so that they can challenge their allocation if it is not. In *Savva* and *KM*, the courts have emphasised the importance of *transparency* by authorities in how they calculate – and check – the value of a personal budget, and in *Savva* the court endorsed transparency regarding the operation of the RAS itself.

The discrepancy between law and policy yawns wide: an indicative budget arrived at by a RAS is not an entitlement – a person has no legal right to a personal budget of that value, only to have their assessed eligible needs met by the local authority. And even if an authority uses a RAS to estimate the value of a personal budget, it will *also* have to conduct some kind of support planning process to check that value is appropriate. It is therefore, *a priori* questionable whether a RAS really can deliver a reduction in local authority bureaucracy in support planning, and whether it can truly divorce itself from subjective judgments by social care practitioners as to the cost of meeting a person's assessed eligible needs.

How RASs work in practice

A small number of empirical studies have examined how RASs work in practice and cast doubt on whether RASs are achieving any of the aims their supporters intended. The Department of Health (DH, 2010c, p 42) has said that the first principle underpinning RASs should be transparency, and this approach has been endorsed by ADASS (2010) and the Court of Appeal in *Savva*. However, a survey of 20 authorities revealed a small number that refused to disclose how their RAS worked – even when a request was made under the Freedom of Information Act 2000 (Series and Clements, 2013).

The basis for these refusals varied. Some authorities were concerned that if service users understood how points were scored and translated into a cash value they might 'game' their responses, a concern that suggests these authorities did not trust service users to self-assess their needs, or did not understand that they retained the legal responsibility for ensuring the accuracy of assessments. One local authority refused to disclose the workings of its RAS because it hoped to market it to other authorities, and if its algorithm were in the public domain it would not be able to profit from selling it. Another was *unable* to disclose how its RAS worked because the local authority had purchased it from a private company and they themselves had no idea how it worked. Eventually – following either adverse publicity or a referral to the Information Commissioner's Office – the authorities who held the information did disclose the workings of their RAS. However, no local authority featured in the study had made efforts to publish its RAS in accordance with the ADASS (2010) guidance, and some were shared in a format that made it extremely difficult to unpick the algorithm used.

This lack of transparency was all the more concerning when it came to how the RASs worked. Of the 20 authorities surveyed, only 13 were still using points-based RASs, and three authorities indicated that they had abandoned points-based RASs due to concerns about their accuracy. When the authors were able to look at raw data themselves, they found the accuracy of RASs to be very low, and it varied between client groups. Some local authorities had given up on points-based RASs and moved to using 'ready reckoners', and some authorities were still using traditional community care assessment practices.

All the points-based RASs were developed by scoring 'live cases' against the needs questionnaire, and then looking at the average cost of meeting needs for people with a particular points profile. So, for example, a RAS could be built on the assumption that a person scoring 16 points would on average have support needs costing £100 per week. The trouble is, these estimates are exactly that – an *average* score. Data obtained by Slasberg and colleagues (2012a), from one of the RAS pilot sites, suggests that the data the RASs were built on could have been very 'noisy' indeed. This data revealed that in only a tiny proportion of cases the RAS was modelled on did the actual cost of meeting a person's needs reflect the average value that the RAS would predict; in some cases, the cost could be as much as *five times more or less* than the value anticipated by the RAS (Slasberg et al, 2012a, p 164). One local authority featured in the Series and Clements study (2013) had reduced this average amount by 15% to produce an indicative amount for its RAS. Even from the outset, it was clear that in many cases the RAS would allocate people much more than they would otherwise receive to meet their assessed eligible needs, and in other cases it would allocate much less. Sometimes this may reflect a levelling out of inequitable distribution, but there is also a clear danger that RASs may leave people with unmet eligible needs or result in inefficient public expenditure.

When the Series and Clements study (2013) looked into the algorithms underpinning the RASs, they came across a number of concerning features in several cases. Some RASs drastically reduced the amount a RAS would allocate if a person lived with family – regardless of how much support their family was willing and able to provide. Others allocated no points for needs that would very likely be eligible for services, such as requiring assistance with eating. Where the authors were able to obtain raw data on indicative and actual personal budgets, they found that in two out of three areas examined people systematically received less than the RAS estimated they should.

The research also disproved another claim regarding RASs – that they would lead to more equitable distribution of resources between different client groups. The authors found that many authorities were using different tariffs for different client groups, which could reflect the differing unit cost of care for the different services they might use. However, they also found that for two of the three authorities using 'universal' RASs, whose processes they could look at in detail, these inequalities remained. In these cases, not only was the RAS itself allocating more to some groups than others – which could simply reflect increased levels of need for these groups – but the *discrepancy* between what the RAS indicated a personal budget should be, and what it actually was, varied significantly between groups. So, for example, people with learning disabilities might in practice receive a few thousand pounds less than the RAS indicated they should, but people with mental health problems or older people might receive *tens* of thousands of pounds less. In effect, these inequalities were creeping back in after the RAS process as authorities decreased entitlements *below* the indicative amount.

Conclusion

RASs occupy a peculiar place in law – they are not required by law, nor do they deliver legally enforceable entitlements, and the courts continue to require local authorities to perform the support planning process that the RAS was supposed to bypass. Their purpose was to increase transparency – yet they are not always publicly available, they can be very complex and difficult to understand, and they may hide unfair assumptions within their very algorithms. They have always been, and often continue to be, inaccurate at predicting the cost of a person's care. This means that authorities relying too much on RASs may under- or over-allocate resources in discharging their legal obligations. Where RASs could have increased resource allocations to client groups who have traditionally been disadvantaged by discretionary community care assessment and planning processes, these increased allocations can be – and are – overridden, to maintain the unfair status quo. Research suggests that self-directed support systems that incorporate RASs do not cut bureaucracy (Slasberg et al, 2012a), which may be because their allocations must still be checked against support plans by local authorities for reasons of fairness and transparency. RASs may be useful for local authorities to *audit* how they are allocating resources, but all the signs suggest they are frequently not achieving any of the aims they were originally designed for, and in some cases may be achieving the very opposite.

FIVE

Safeguarding, risk and personalisation

Jill Manthorpe

In Chapter Two, Catherine Needham and Jon Glasby observe that 'attitudes to risk and expectations of the state are essentially contested and yet are crucial to the deployment of social care policies' (p 24). This chapter takes this observation further by interweaving the narratives of personalisation, risk and safeguarding. It draws on a set of research studies in which the implications of personalisation, risk and safeguarding have been debated. The studies include the evaluation of the individual budget pilots (Manthorpe et al, 2009, 2011), the evaluation of the test sites of self-directed support in Scotland (Hunter et al, 2012) and a study of the implementation of the Mental Capacity Act 2005 and its interface with safeguarding policy and practice that was undertaken with the Alzheimer's Society (Manthorpe and Samsi, 2013). The context of these studies is also influenced by work on dementia and risk that was published as a set of guidance by the Department of Health, entitled *Nothing ventured, nothing gained* (Manthorpe and Moriarty, 2010) and on the Making Safeguarding Personal programme of practice development in the social care sector (see Klee and Williams, 2013; Manthorpe et al, 2014).

As a prelude to the chapter, this introduction briefly outlines what is meant by the term 'safeguarding' in the English context (in Scotland the term 'adult protection' is more commonly used [Johnson, 2012]). The term 'adult safeguarding' has a precise focus in social policy in England, being mainly used to describe the systems in place whereby public policy legitimates protection and enhances the human rights of vulnerable adults or adults at risk. Critiques of these concepts abound, such as the vagueness of the term 'at risk' (being at risk of what precisely?); whether the term 'vulnerable adults' focuses unduly on individual disability, frailty or impairment; whether the underlying values are paternal or over-protective; whether such terms minimise criminal activity as mistreatment or poor practice (Dixon et al, 2010) and thus deny victims access to justice (Dunn et al, 2008); or if such terms unduly focus on individual perpetrators rather than vulnerable situations or contexts (Burns et al, 2013).

This leads to observations on a second definitional debate around the specific term 'risk'. This has become an over-stretched or elastic noun. Risk may be defined as the likelihood or probability of an event occurring. As a result, risk assessment and risk management are inevitably matters of calculation and must involve some element of uncertainty. In the UK, the terms 'risk enablement' or 'positive risk taking' have been coined to focus on the idea that the process of measuring or calculating risk involves balancing the positive benefits from taking risks against the negative effects of attempting to avoid risk altogether. This is in response to what the Nuffield Council on Bioethics (2009), in its report on dementia, portrayed as a risk assessment approach that concentrates on minimising or eliminating risk without considering what opportunities and benefits are thereby forgone. The Council favoured the term 'risk–benefit assessment' to emphasise the importance of taking into account the wellbeing and autonomy of the person with dementia, as well as their need for protection from physical harm. Such approaches may be more widely applied.

There are many connections between terms such as risk enablement, risk–benefit analysis, and positive risk management, so much so that they seem to be used interchangeably. Currently, they are commonly encountered in professional circles, so although people generally weigh up advantages and disadvantages when assessing risk, they may not actually use these exact words to describe what they do or the calculations they employ. The Dementia Risk Guidance illustrated this balancing act when talking of the risk of a person with dementia getting lost or harmed if they went out unaccompanied but suggesting the hazard might need to be considered in the light of other possible risks of boredom and frustration from remaining inside and the potential gains from exercise and social contact (Manthorpe and Moriarty, 2010).

As this chapter aims to outline, many of these debates about the nature of safeguarding and of risk can be discerned in the narratives of personalisation (Needham, 2011a). For example, Sarah Carr (2010, p 55) suggested that one indication of a supportive social care system would be how it incorporates self-directed support with safeguarding policy and practice. She suggested that training on how to detect abuse and the enablement of risk should be offered to both staff and people using services, particularly those taking up personal budgets, although there is very little evidence of what effective training might look like. As this chapter will show, Carr's (2010) recommendation that practitioners need to be supported by local authorities to incorporate safeguarding and risk enablement into relationship-based, person-centred working would also have to take on board one of the key tenets of risk enablement – that things will indeed go wrong at times (otherwise it is not a risk but a certainty).

Early days

The narratives of personalisation in social care services were profoundly informed by the results of the evaluation of the individual budget (IB) pilots (see Glendinning et al, 2008), as other chapters in this book identify. As part of this evaluation, the authors described the approach to adult safeguarding taken in the 13 pilot sites during the pilot phase of IBs and explored the interface between adult protection and safeguarding. Fieldwork took the form of qualitative interviews carried out in 2007. The participants were all the IB sites' adult safeguarding co-ordinators (ASCs) (the generic term for the local authority lead managers with responsibility for adult safeguarding). In a first round of interviews, ASCs reported simultaneous pressures for greater user choice and control in social care and for greater user safety and public reassurances. The ASCs had not been informed of the IB developments and their lack of involvement with IB changes was possibly generously attributed to the rapid pace of change in the local authority pilot areas amid a feeling that IBs might also be an experiment that could have been curtailed. The ASCs felt that their knowledge of adult protection systems and processes were not used in IB implementation and so their wealth of experience in adult safeguarding and managing concerns about direct payments was not drawn upon.

Converging

The second round of interviews with ASCs as part of the evaluation of the IB pilots took place in 2008 (Manthorpe et al, 2011). While participants recognised the potential benefits of IBs, their concerns had not been assuaged about the potential for overlooking the risks of abuse and exploitation. IBs in the form of direct payments were generally acknowledged to carry greater risks than care-managed services, partly because it was emerging that legislation aimed at barring unsuitable workers (the Protection of Vulnerable Adults [POVA] list under the Care Standards Act 2000; its successor under the Safeguarding Vulnerable Groups Act 2006; and currently through the Disclosure and Barring Service under the Protection of Freedoms Act 2012) did not cover self-employed people or family members working as personal assistants. In addition, ASCs reported that criminal record checks were not being routinely conducted because IB holders were permitted to decline to do so; indeed, they might be deterred from doing so because of the trouble and expense (this situation is not permitted in Scotland). Several pointed to the risks of the rise in casual employment situations typical among personal assistants:

> 'There's a high-risk situation here but I am very supportive of IBs – I would not want this to have a negative impact. We should have very clear strategies and manage the risk and help people on IBs.' (ASC12)

Many of these workers are hard to reach (Dixon et al, 2013) and as Christensen and Manthorpe (in press) have found, some of them are 'under the radar', being recruited abroad and being told to avoid officialdom. Similarly, ASCs expressed fears that people determined to abuse would target IB holders to exploit them:

> 'My views haven't altered – they have only been strengthened.... I don't think we've done enough in this field. These people [abusers] work in clusters and associates. It will become known that this group is ripe for targeting.' (ASC5)

Participants were also alert to the potential for IBs to destabilise family relationships and they argued that this needed to be addressed:

> 'I think a more general point – in those situations whether a service user employs a friend or family member – services need to be cautious about the dynamics – about how the service user is receiving IB – their overall autonomy and independence. Because, again, you are talking about relationships that go beyond – "I pay you" to personal relationships.... The danger doing this job is that you have a fairly jaundiced view of humanity really.' (ASC7)

However, the ASCs' knowledge and experiences were beginning to be used by their colleagues in some areas, in dealing with specific problems and in shaping channels of communication. In some sites, the largely separated discourses of protection and empowerment were starting to converge. Nonetheless, many of the debates remained on parallel tracks and were articulated nationally in the consultation undertaken for the review of *No secrets* (DH, 2009a). The study concluded that aspects of safeguarding needed to be built into personalisation including regular and respectful contact between those responsible for managing the transformation of adult services and their colleagues in adult safeguarding. It was evident that the latter were rarely involved in training, risk assessment and risk management about IBs and their successors, personal budgets, particularly in the form of direct payments. In response to the IB evaluation and other expressed concerns, the Department of Health (2010d) issued its first report on the linkages between safeguarding and personalisation, summarising legal responsibilities that had not been clear previously.

Border crossing

As Hunter and colleagues (2012) noted, there were marked similarities in the findings of the evaluations of the self-directed support (SDS) test sites in Scotland and those of the IB pilots in England (Glendinning et al, 2008). Both found that adult safeguarding issues had not been initially considered. There appeared to have been no learning from the IBs' experiences in the later Scottish experiments. More specific to Scotland, the adult protection leads (APLs) in Scotland thought that the SDS policy had not engaged with the implications of the Adult Support and Protection (Scotland) Act (2007), which gives greater powers of entry and intervention than in England. It appeared that APLs seemed to have been 'by-standers' in the implementation of SDS in Scotland and consideration of linkages between adult protection and SDS in the test sites seemed embryonic. The APLs were aware that the aspirations of SDS went beyond the confines of direct payments but did not appear to help fashion these aspirations. These could include contributing to managing the risks of abuse of SDS funds by recipients on the one hand and the risks, on the other hand, that they might be at risk of being abused. Hunter and colleagues (2012) concluded that some of the debates about risk and safeguarding were becoming entangled. Concerns by local authority managers or politicians about the use and misuse of public funds might also overlap with fears about potential exploitation of adults at risk of harm.

This study illustrated how the debate over risk and personalisation may cover a myriad of perceptions of risk and of abuse. An adult at risk, for example, could be abusing the system, but could also be being exploited. To minimise such risks, professionals have been reminded that in the case of personal health budgets (PHBs) there are ways to minimise temptation or financial unruliness:

For example, PHBs can be held by a third party rather than being directly paid to individuals in the form of a direct payment to increase financial control. This may be appropriate where individuals have, for example, serious addiction issues. (Alakeson and Perkins, 2012, p 10)

Managing risks

These early observations from the IB evaluation and the SDS test site evaluation were followed by other developments affecting the transformation process of personalisation. These include the Mental Capacity Act (MCA) 2005 in England and Wales and the later changes to regulations permitting 'proxy' personal budgets – held, for example, by relatives where a person lacks decision-making capacity (for example, they have severe dementia or severe learning disabilities) (DH, 2009b). Interestingly, much of the detail of local implementation of the MCA was to fall on safeguarding teams or lead officers (ASCs), who generally took on this area of policy and practice for the local authority. Thus their potential role in advising on personal budgets procedures and cases increased as they were most familiar with the MCA provisions, such as Best Interests decision-making processes and the obligations imposed by the MCA on those caring for people lacking mental capacity, including the criminalisation of ill treatment and wilful neglect.

In some areas, but not many, structures such as risk enablement panels were established (see, for example, London Borough of Newham, 2009; DH, 2010d), but in many local areas it appears that decision-making panels to approve or sign off a personal budget focus more on the cost-effectiveness of the planned budget or become overwhelmed by having to agree to risk calculations and the inevitable elements of uncertainty:

> This seems to be playing out differently in different parts of the country, but there is a risk that some of the 'risk enablement panels' that are being set up to support personal budget holders and staff to take positive risks, could actually become too slow and risk-averse – leading to a re-bureaucratisation of the system. (Glasby, 2012b, p 16)

In 2009 the system of direct payments was extended to include those who lack the capacity to consent to receiving them. The guidance (DH/DCSF, 2009) accompanying these regulations explains how direct payments services should be developed locally, how issues of consent, capacity and ability to manage should be approached and how direct payments should be used. It explains where additional support is required and available, and describes the monitoring and review process. It also includes a section on troubleshooting or managing specific risks. While devising a support plan is one thing, we know little about how best to monitor plans and their outcomes, so that aspirations for greater choice and control do not just remain on paper.

Research has yet to collect and analyse whether support plans agreed around personal budgets outcomes are integrated with adult safeguarding plans (devised, for instance, following an investigation and case conclusion whether the allegation of abuse or neglect is substantiated or not). Our current study is investigating this question (www.kcl.ac.uk/sspp/kpi/scwru/res/knowledge/risks.aspx).

Capacity concerns

The relevance of the MCA to personal budgets, particularly direct payments, emerged slowly (Alzheimer's Society, 2011a) but rights to safeguarding were better articulated. In an interview-based study that focused on the provisions of the MCA, 15 ASCs were asked whether they thought the move to personal budgets/self-directed support might affect the likelihood of financial abuse among people with memory problems, cognitive impairment or dementia, and how safeguarding services could assist in reducing any risks (Manthorpe and Samsi, 2013). Practitioners working with people with dementia were also asked to identify financial abuse indicators and patterns more generally among people with dementia (see Manthorpe et al, 2014), which drew attention to the problems facing people with early and mild dementia, as well as those with more severe or distressing symptoms, in making judgements over money and possibly being over-trusting.

In relation to the history of abuse and exploitation of people with dementia, perhaps no professional knows better than ASCs of the risks of inflexible, poor quality, unreliable social care support where people with dementia and their carers have traditionally had little choice and control over quality and outcomes. They have witnessed the 'inherent risks' of such care and support services that do not always meet people's needs and sometimes are abusive and neglectful. However, it is not just care workers and professionals that may be abusive; in practice, ASCs also encounter family carers who perpetrate neglect and abuse, and, outside the social and healthcare arenas, they are aware of the targeting of people with dementia by those with criminal intent. One key finding of this study (Samsi et al, 2014) was that a polarised view of standard services as 'inherently risky' and of personal budgets as 'safer' holds little water. But many ASCs remain concerned that the interactions between personalisation and safeguarding have not been thought about sufficiently and that the safeguards of the MCA do not apply widely. Samsi and colleagues argued that if their concerns are not assuaged this may exacerbate their perceptions that efforts in protection are naively associated with pessimism about personal budgets.

Making Safeguarding Personal

More recently, others have also explored how broader aspects of personalisation – greater independence, choice and control – could be built into safeguarding activities and the Local Government Association has worked on a sector-led improvement programme entitled Making Safeguarding Personal (MSP) (see Klee and Williams, 2013). This development project was set up in response to concerns from some safeguarding stakeholders and practitioners in England that the focus on process and procedure in adult safeguarding had become too 'impersonal'. As an alternative to processes that might not be person-centred, personalisation offered a framework that concentrated on the desired outcomes of the individual concerned. The first MSP project aimed to explore the potential for new or under-used approaches to adult safeguarding practice.

The first programme also encouraged an outcomes focus and urged practitioners to consider a wide range of responses to the circumstances of people at risk whose lives were being negatively affected by abuse and neglect. As the MSP programme is taking place at a time of financial pressures and local reorganisations, this is challenging. The context is further complicated by predicted changes following the Care Act 2014 that will place adult safeguarding on a firmer footing through statutory recognition of Safeguarding Adults Boards and will set up a duty for councils to make enquiries where safeguarding concerns are raised. This will enhance the priority given to adult safeguarding by councils, the NHS, police and other organisations. However, the 'culture' of adult safeguarding is not fully understood and its values are not as well articulated as other forms of practice. This makes it difficult when engaging with the highly charged culture of personalisation within which the rhetoric of choice, empowerment, 'light-touch' regulation and monitoring are frequently voiced. It is easy perhaps for safeguarding to be seen as risk-averse, paternalistic and process-driven.

Conclusion

As the early studies of personalisation in England and self-directed support in Scotland have exposed (Manthorpe et al, 2009, 2011; Hunter et al, 2012; Samsi et al, 2014), relationships between personalisation and safeguarding are being belatedly constructed at practice and at policy level so that the two aspirations become more compatible. However, statutory local authority adult services are only one sector where personalisation is a policy goal – there is currently commitment in the NHS to personal health budgets (see Part Four) and to extend personal budgets to promote mental health recovery (Alakeson and Perkins, 2012). Cultural change is seen as part of the way in which healthcare professionals can 'deliver' necessary advice and support for patients and their families. They too need to ensure that adults at risk are not exposed to undue harm or encounter risks of harm without support. The lesson from social care is that safeguarding and personalisation need to be both informed by risk – and that they should be both sides of the same coin rather than different currencies.

Acknowledgments and disclaimer

This chapter is based on background work undertaken as part of the Social Care Workforce Research Unit's work for the Policy Research Programme of the Department of Health. The views are those of the author and should not be interpreted as necessarily those of the Department of Health.

SIX

Can personalisation work for older people?

Liz Lloyd

Introduction

The debates and controversies surrounding the personalisation agenda that have already been identified in this text are clearly evident in the context of services for older people. The development of any policy can be understood as a battle of ideas in which there will be winners and losers (Colebatch, 2005). In this case, as Needham (2011b) has pointed out, the personalisation agenda has gained enormous popularity in the field of social care policy, having now become effectively 'the only game in town'. However, the ambiguous nature of the concept effectively means that the battle of ideas is still continuing. On the one hand, personalisation is characterised as a revolution in social care, a wholesale cultural shift in the perceptions about how people who need support should be able to exercise control over how it is given. On the other, it is more prosaically seen in terms of the levels of implementation of personal budgets (PBs) and direct payments (DPs) to individual service users, which redistributes responsibility from the state to individuals. Since services for older people constitute more than half of social services expenditure (HSCIC, 2012), it is unsurprising that much attention is being paid to the implementation of personalisation in this sphere, although older service users appear to be less enthusiastic than others about PBs and DPs (Glendinning et al, 2008; Hatton and Waters, 2011). The pressure on councils to increase their uptake raises questions about whether older people are also under pressure to accept PBs or DPs, thus undermining the claims to increased choice and control that are made for them.

This chapter will examine the unfolding story of personalisation in the context of social care services for older people. Ageing is a crucially important issue at both macro- and micro-levels of service provision and the discussion will consider the impact of societal ageing on the development of policies as well as the advantages and disadvantages of personalisation for older service users. The main strands of contemporary critiques of personalisation all have a bearing on this discussion. In general terms, these critiques focus on the willingness and capability of local authorities and the professionals that work in them to implement personalisation policies in daily practice, particularly in the context of the current economic circumstances. There is also the view (as outlined by Needham and Glasby in this volume) that personalisation is a 'Trojan horse' for the imposition of neoliberal policies. Another critique is that the personalisation agenda has been shaped by younger disabled adults whose demands differ from those of older people (Lloyd, 2010).

The discussion will take a broad view of the personalisation agenda, in order to make sense of the competing perspectives that exist in the context of social care for older people. For example, the view that personalisation could enable councils to concentrate their diminishing resources on a smaller, more needful group of older people (Audit Commission, 2010) contrasts with the view that the priority for councils is to take action on current high levels of unmet need among older people (Humphries et al, 2010; AgeUK, 2011). These competing perspectives over service priorities have major implications for older people who need help and support. Moreover, these priorities have arisen not only from recent economic crises, but also from demographic trends over decades. Ageing and personalisation are, therefore, interrelated in complex ways.

Demographic trends and the cost of care

Increased life expectancy has been one of the most dramatic social changes of the past century and demographic trends have been portrayed imaginatively as a 'grey tsunami' or demographic 'time bomb'. These images form the cultural backdrop to the personalisation of services and create a particular, age-related, set of concerns about social care. As age dependency ratios shift and projections of increasing demand for health and social care services are calculated, the sense of urgency in policies is intense. The first report of the Select Committee on Public Service and Demographic Change, *Are we ready for ageing?*, concluded that as a country the UK is 'woefully unprepared' for the ageing of the population and that by 2022 an increase in public expenditure of 37% on 2010 figures would be necessary for social care and Continuing Healthcare 'to keep pace with expected demographic and unit cost pressures' (House of Lords, 2013, para 23).

It is important to emphasise that although older people's services represent over half of the local authorities' expenditure on social care, overall levels of spending on social care for all adults amount to just 1.6% of GDP and spending on social care is a small proportion of overall spending on services for older people – around 6% in 2010-11 (Charlesworth and Thorlby, 2012). An equally important point is that only a minority of older people use social care services – around 15%, according to the Audit Commission (2010). The common practice of juxtaposing current use of services by older people against demographic trends in order to make projections about increased demand is open to criticism. Falkingham and colleagues (2010), for example, make the pertinent point that there is a need to disaggregate the data on age groups rather than treating older people as a homogeneous group. Those who are oldest tend to be most likely to need social care services as a result of health problems. Between the ages of 65 and 74, less than 10% of people have a 'serious disability' compared with around 33% of men and 42% of women aged 85 and over. The projected increase in numbers of people in the oldest age groups is presented as part of the case for change in the White Paper, *Caring for our future*:

> By 2030, population estimates show the number of people aged over 85 will be almost twice what it is now, and there will be 59,000 people aged over 100 – five times as many as there are today. Over the next 30 years, the number of people living with dementia is projected to double. (HM Government, 2012, p 16)

There are also social factors to take into account. For example, the number of people in private households who live alone rises sharply with age, amounting to just under half of men and two-thirds of women aged 85 and over compared with less than a quarter of men and less than a half of women aged 65 and over (Falkingham et al, 2010). When gender, ethnicity, socioeconomic status and other social factors are also taken into account, it is evident that older people are an extremely heterogeneous group. Variations at the individual level add significantly to the complexity. It is neither possible nor desirable to draw conclusions about an individual person's needs based on their social or economic status. Individual characteristics developed over the life course as well as personal resources all have a major impact on needs in later life and on personal preferences about how these are met.

Of course, achieving this kind of variation is precisely what the broad personalisation agenda is about and there are many reasons therefore to regard a more person-centred approach to support and care as a boon to older people. However, a major problem arises as the ideals of person-centred, individually tailored services collide with the priority of keeping a grip on spending because of societal ageing. Common strategies used by local authorities to control costs have been to tighten eligibility criteria to reduce the numbers of people in the system and to impose charges on individual service users. Over recent years, there has been a severe reduction in the range of support available to older people, which follows a more gradual trend in this direction. Indeed, the reduction in numbers of service users who receive a narrower range of services has become an accepted outcome of community care policies since the 1990s. Depending on one's point of view, these developments can be interpreted as successful management of scarce resources or as failure to meet need. Either way, there are serious implications for personalisation. There is a major problem, therefore, in promoting more individualised forms of service provision for older people when en masse they are regarded as an economic problem for service providers and policymakers.

There is no clear consensus on the potential of PBs and DPs to save money (Slay, 2010). They are regarded by the Association of Directors of Adult Social Services and the Department of Health as 'cost-neutral'. A cost-benefit analysis carried out by Woolham and Benton (2012) identified poorer outcomes for older people than other age groups. The *Caring for our future* White Paper presents personalisation as having the potential to improve value for money rather than to cut costs. There is, however, also wide acknowledgement that older people who are already eligible for services do not receive them and that there are many others who need assistance to stop them from declining further (Humphries et al, 2010). Given the policy trends discussed earlier, it is highly unlikely that the scope of social care services will widen to embrace currently unmet needs among older people. There is also increasing recognition that there is little chance of making savings that do not affect frontline services, because the quest for greater efficiencies in social care has been occurring over several years (Charlesworth and Thorlby, 2012). It follows that, at present, cost neutrality is a wholly inadequate basis on which to reform services provision.

Needham's point about the ambiguity that exists concerning the meaning of personalisation and the language of reform is relevant here (Needham, 2011a). The personalisation agenda has provided a convenient rationale for actions such as the closure of day centres and the sale of care homes. There is an irreconcilable tension within the policy process when individuals are encouraged to take control over organising their own care and support when managers of social care services are striving to maximise efficiency and reduce service costs as much as possible. Reductions in the level of resources within personal budgets are to be expected, despite evidence that unless the level of the budget is set higher than that needed for basic help there will be no increase in the flexibility for individuals in organising support (Glendinning et al, 2008; Woolham and Benton, 2012). In addition, lower levels of resources will undoubtedly be reflected in worse pay and conditions for support workers as well as increased pressure on families to provide more care than would have been expected. There are, therefore, good reasons to be cautious about policies and practices on personalisation as applied to older people. To bring about change in older people's care and support, local authorities would need to do much more than simply delegate responsibility for cost savings to older people through inadequately resourced PBs and DPs.

The preventive capacity of personalisation

The preventive potential of personalisation is important to consider at this point. The vision for care and support set out in the *Caring for our future* White Paper (HM Government, 2012) is to enable people to stay 'active, connected and independent' and the emphasis is on action 'upstream' in order to transform services from being downstream, reactive and crisis-driven. This shift of emphasis could go some way to meeting the demands of Age UK and others for attention to unmet need. In their report on prevention and personalisation, Hudson and Henwood (2008) comment that there is no consensus on the meaning of prevention and that in the context of older people's social care and the focus on people in greatest need it has come to mean keeping them out of institutional care. However, demand for care home places remains steady and is predicted to rise, suggesting that care homes remain an important option for older people. Indeed, the core values of choice and control would support this.

Given the ambiguous meanings of both terms, the association between personalisation and prevention merits careful consideration. In their evaluation of the preventive approaches demonstrated in the Partnership for Older People's Projects, Windle and colleagues (2009) identified that prevention and early intervention can 'work' for older people and help to reduce demand on secondary services, provided they are appropriately funded and managed. This echoes findings from earlier studies that point to the value to older people's health and wellbeing of a little bit of help (Clark et al, 1998) and from community-based projects that promote activity and social inclusion (Teater and Baldwin, 2012; Tulle and Dorrer, 2012). However, there is growing evidence that current financial pressures have led to cuts to projects, thus undermining the potential for building up preventive services (Deeming, 2009). There is therefore a problem inherent in the current policy context, in that while the value of community-based services is increasingly recognised, the ability of organisations to continue providing them has diminished. The closure of day centres is a case in point. Day centres are often characterised as an 'old fashioned' and institutionalised form of service but this view ignores their preventive potential as well as their variety and capacity to adapt to new conditions, including the increased levels of disability and cognitive impairment of the people who attend (Fawcett, 2012). All in all, the evidence suggests that a range of community-based provisions is necessary to the success of the preventive agenda, which can benefit older people's health and wellbeing and promote their social inclusion. As Ellis (2013) argues, there is a different view of community development in the *Caring for our future* White Paper, which is more about the stimulation of a low-cost market for individual PB and DP holders to tap into in order to minimise their reliance on publicly funded provision. In this sense, promoting older people's health and activity levels can be understood as a means to an end, rather than an end in itself.

Ageing, dependency and the need for care

A core, specifically age-related point about the personalisation agenda concerns the capacity of service users to engage in the agenda. In policies, both preventive and personalisation agendas portray an image of an engaged and active consumer citizen who is in charge of their destiny and able to manage their own care. This perspective has been the subject of criticism from a range of perspectives. Scourfield (2007) and Clarke and colleagues (2007) argue that it is a form of abandonment of collective responsibility. Feminist ethicists argue that we should all be understood as individuals with rights and responsibilities but that our individual identities are the *outcome of* our social nature, not *prior to* it (Barnes, 2012). Our social nature reinforces the point that dependency on others is a normal aspect of life, as is our need to give care and support to others. Drawing on her experience as the mother of a disabled child, the feminist ethicist Eva Kittay developed the concept of 'nested dependencies' to describe the way that individuals who require support and care are helped by others who, in turn, benefit from support and care (Kittay, 2002). The help provided by families is enhanced by the input of specialist support from professionals and paid carers, which is also enhanced by good employment practices that do not exploit them. This perspective on networks of care and support might be seen as consistent with some versions of personalisation in which individuals are assisted to find ways of meeting their needs that recognise their relationships with others. However, Barnes (2012) argues strongly that personalisation policies ignore the social, economic and political conditions that shape and influence need and are wholly inconsistent with an ethic of care.

In the White Paper, the need for care and support is presented as something that '76% of older people' will need at some point in later life. The point is made that care affects us all because 'we will all know someone who needs some extra care or support to lead a full and active life' (HM Government, 2012 , p 14). What is meant by a full and active life is not spelt out, but in relation to old age, it needs to be recognised that aspirations for a full and active life change dramatically, as a result of advancing years and declining health (Venn and Arber, 2011; Lloyd et al, 2012). Indeed, it is unquestionably the case that 100% of us will need care and support at some point in our lives and nowadays the likelihood is that this will be in old age when health begins to fail and the end of life draws nearer. Over the past century, there has been an ageing of mortality. Death and dying have become increasingly concentrated in later life, so that the relatively even spread of deaths across different age groups characteristic of the early 1900s has changed dramatically and now around 85% of deaths of males and more than 90% of deaths of females occur over the age of 60. What is more, since 1980 the percentage of deaths among those aged 80 years and over has risen from 21% for males and 43% for females to 43% for males and 62% for females (ONS, 2012). These trends are relevant and important to the personalisation debate. Typically, the health problems experienced in old age are long-term, progressive and complex, involving several conditions. As health declines, it often becomes difficult to assess whether an individual is 'dying from' or 'living with' their health conditions. Nicholson and colleagues (2012) describe the deaths of older people as an 'uncertain and dwindling process'. The ageing of mortality also means that bereavement and widowhood are common in old age. In these circumstances, daily life for an individual older person can be very demanding indeed as well as precarious and unpredictable, creating a need for particular kinds of support, protection and care (Lloyd et al, 2012).

Questions therefore arise about the way that the personalisation agenda has been conceptualised and implemented in practice. For example, the claim that service users are the experts in their own lives is open to question in the context of the crisis and shock that often accompanies the loss of mobility or bereavement. Although the circumstances of older people are relatively common within their age group, individual older people do not 'know' how to manage the changes they experience. This is not to suggest that older people should be passive recipients of professionally organised care, but to stress the importance of thinking more broadly about the meaning of terms such as independence, choice and control, and about the way these are used in policies to construct a particular version of citizenship. Lloyd and colleagues (2012) outlined the reflexive process described by older research participants as they came to terms with the need to adjust to their unstable and changing circumstances while also striving to maintain their health and independence as much as possible. This process was helped greatly by the presence of supportive family or friends as well as by professionals whose sensitivity and attentiveness enabled the older person to make decisions and adapt their way of living. This process can be understood as the exercise of choice and control but not as portrayed in policies. From this perspective, older people's apparent reluctance to choose DPs can be understood somewhat differently. In policy debates, the tendency is to identify ways of breaking down the barriers to their uptake, which are regarded as arising from organisational procedures or professional resistance.

The development of managed PBs was designed specifically to enable an individual to have more or less support with organising their care. They have been criticised as offering a less liberating form of personalisation than DPs. However, there are reasons to see the possibility of improved support for older people through managed PBs. As Newbronner and colleagues (2011) identified in their review of PB implementation in local authorities, support is crucial to success from the perspective of both older service users and their carers. Importantly, the authors found that this support was best provided in the form of individual, face-to-face attention from a practitioner with whom the service users and carers had built up a relationship. The problem is that the tightening of eligibility criteria discussed earlier has normalised a narrow and impoverished perception of need in old age. What this has increasingly come to mean for many, especially those living alone, is the restriction of services to help with basic personal care and hygiene, meal preparation and medication. Staffing costs are crucial to a manager's calculations and the amount of time practitioners have to spend with older people has been reduced to the bare minimum, making it harder for them to provide the kind of person-centred support that Newbronner and colleagues (2011) highlighted. In addition, as Newbronner and colleagues pointed out, the time professionals spent with older people enabled them to change their care arrangements as their health conditions fluctuated.

The social and cultural backdrop of service provision discussed above is important to bear in mind. Ageist views about the burdensomeness of older people who are unable to care for themselves, together with the portrayal of unsustainable pressure on resources as a result of their increasing numbers, are reflected in the language of policies and influence daily practice in health and social care organisations. It is unsurprising that policymakers give priority to macro-economic concerns but policies on support for older people are made with little or no reference to the daily practices of care (Twigg, 2006) except when a scandal erupts and care practices come under scrutiny. Importantly, ageist assumptions influence not only the decisions made by managers and practitioners, but also those made by older people about whether or not to seek help, for both practical and moral reasons. Older people, particularly those from minority groups, might not know about services, they might doubt that they would qualify for a service and they also might question whether they merit help. In the study by Lloyd and colleagues (2012) referred to earlier, participants set a high value on being seen by others to be independent, although what independence meant to them was variable. For some, caring within the family meant having their independence preserved, while for others the purchase of services such as house cleaning and private transport had the same meaning. These variations underline the importance of relationships that enable individuality to be preserved.

Conclusion

The current context of older people's services cannot be said to be conducive to person-centred care. Indeed, the shortage of resources within the care system is a serious stumbling-block. Moreover, the priority given to the implementation of budgets misses the point about the need for a broader range of supportive relationships. The ethic of care proposed by feminist ethicists does not consign older people to a category of passive objects of care, nor does it rely on older service users or their carers having become savvy consumers. It regards care as a necessity for all that should be provided in a way that is responsive to each. The evidence discussed in this chapter suggests that efforts to increase the uptake of DPs and PBs are a distraction from wider concerns about the direction of policies on social care for older people, while well-resourced person-centred support from families, community organisations and professionals is a vital means of securing older people's social inclusion and wellbeing.

SEVEN

Personalisation: where do carers fit?

Wendy Mitchell, Jenni Brooks and Caroline Glendinning

Introduction

Adult social care in England prioritises personalisation for service users of the support they receive (DH, 2005, 2007). Personalisation is founded on arguments about promoting choice, control and empowerment of individual service users. Individuals are conceptualised as active consumers of public services, able to exercise enhanced choice over how their needs should be met, thus experiencing greater control over their own lives. However, these arguments appear to ignore the realities of older and disabled people's lives, which are often embedded in networks of support from close kin and friends.

Carers, especially family carers, play important supporting roles in the lives of many older and disabled people. Among developed welfare states England is unusual, as carers have secured rights to assessments of their needs. Carers can also receive services (or cash grants) as well as an income replacement benefit (Carers Allowance) to support their care-giving roles (Carers [Recognition and Services] Act, 1995; Carers [Equal Opportunities] Act, 2004; HM Government, 2008). However, the arguments and assumptions underpinning personalisation – that this will promote choice, control and empowerment – appear to overlook the perspectives of carers. Arksey and Glendinning (2007), in a review of research evidence on choice and care giving, drew attention to the relative invisibility of carers in a series of policy statements on personalisation in adult social care and concluded that choice remains highly problematic for carers. Indeed, choice making is a complex process as people do not make choices in social isolation; choice making frequently involves weighing up options with others, often carers (Mitchell, 2012). However, policy and practice both reflect a widespread tendency to overlook the complex dynamics of care-giving relationships and conflate the needs and aspirations of carers and the people they support into a single (implicitly harmonious) unit. The interdependencies that often exist between disabled and older people and the relatives and friends who support them (Fine and Glendinning, 2005; Kröger, 2009) are also widely overlooked. Thus, the services and support provided to disabled or older people can have important benefits for carers too (Pickard, 2004). This impact can be both direct, where services for the disabled or older person, such as day or respite care, benefit carers by giving them a break; and indirect, if, for example, carers derive satisfaction from knowing the person they support receives appropriate, good-quality services.

Carers have received relatively little attention in the growing body of research on personalisation (Flynn, 2005; Jones et al, 2012; Moran et al, 2012). This marginalisation appears inconsistent with the public recognition and policy initiatives raising the profile of carers and their needs over the past 15 years (HM Government, 2008; Carers UK, 2010; DH, 2010e). English policy and practice is further complicated by ongoing debates between the disability and carers' movements, particularly questions about whether policies that support carers perpetuate disabled and older people's dependence (Shakespeare, 2000). This chapter explores the challenges and potential tensions adult social care faces arising from this dislocation between personalisation and carer policies and practice.

Background

As mentioned earlier, carers have legal rights. In 1995, carers gained entitlement to an assessment of their own needs (Carers [Recognition and Services] Act). This right was extended in 2000 (Disabled Children Act) to entitlement to a carer assessment even if the person they supported refused or was ineligible for local authority support. The 2004 Carers (Equal Opportunities) Act placed a statutory duty on local authorities to inform people (with regular and substantial care responsibilities) of their right to separate assessments, in which carers' aspirations for employment, learning and leisure should be considered. Since 2000, carers have also been able to receive cash direct payments in their own right. The revised national carers' strategy included a commitment that everyone using adult social care, including carers, should be able to receive a personal budget (PB) (HM Government, 2010). However, in 2009-10, only 4% of carers reported having been assessed (Princess Royal Trust for Carers and Crossroads Care, 2010) and by March 2012 only 51,191 carers reported receipt of a PB.

Research into the impacts of direct payments has found that carers face additional responsibilities, such as recruiting and employing paid care workers (Carers UK, 2008; Grootegoed et al, 2010). However, these additional responsibilities could be offset by benefits for carers. For example, increasing independence for the disabled or older person could facilitate opportunities for carers to reduce their caring responsibilities. The national evaluation of the individual budget (IB) pilot projects in England compared carers of IB recipients with carers of people receiving conventional social care support (Glendinning et al, 2008). Carers of IB recipients were often involved in managing the disabled or older person's IB and coordinating her/his support arrangements. These carers spent more time on care-related activities than carers of people using conventional services. Despite this, outcomes were better for carers of IB recipients, who also reported IB support planning processes as more holistic than traditional service user assessments. Hence, support planning could be an indicator of positive outcomes for carers (Glendinning et al, 2009; Jones et al, 2012; Moran et al, 2012; see also TLAP, 2013a).

The evaluation of personal health budgets (PHBs) also found that carers providing assistance to individuals receiving PHBs were more likely to report better quality of life and perceived health compared with carers assisting an individual in the control group. Carers in the PHB group also generally reported less impact of care giving on their health (Forder et al, 2012). Furthermore, qualitative interviews with a small sample of carers of PHB holders found the potential for both direct and indirect benefits from PHBs for carers (Davidson et al, 2012).

The IB evaluation also demonstrated how the introduction of personalisation occurred, at least initially, with little consideration of, or coordination with, local authority responsibilities towards carers. The IB evaluation found no explicit reference to how carers should be included in IBs and few local authority carer lead officers played an active role in the introduction of IBs (Moran et al, 2012). Some localities had included only limited prompts or questions about carers' circumstances and needs in their new IB assessment processes. Variation was also apparent among the IB pilot sites in how help provided by family carers was treated in the disabled/older person's assessment and in calculating the level of the service user's IB. There were also inconsistencies in the roles practitioners expected carers to play in helping IB holders plan and manage their IB. These inconsistencies suggest that the failure to consider carers in the implementation of personal budgets is an important design flaw within personalisation.

Research commissioned by Carers UK has also identified considerable variability in how (self-) assessment forms for PBs consider carers' needs (Clements et al, 2009). Local authorities have been reminded, as they implement personalisation, of their obligations to adhere to legislation and practice on supporting carers (CSCI, 2008a; SCIE in conjunction with Carers UK, 2009). The Law Commission (2008) has also recognised this disconnection between personalisation and carers' policies and has proposed that the legal framework for the provision of services to carers and its relationship to that of service users should be reviewed. The outcome of this review is reflected in the Care Act 2014, which places carers' rights to public support on an equal footing with the rights of the person they support.

Official guidance (DH, 2010e) recommends that service user assessments for personal budgets should routinely ask carers how much help they are willing and able to give. Separate assessments of carers' needs and those of service users should be coordinated, so that information from both assessments can be brought together to inform support planning. Indicative budgets for service users should take into account the availability and level of support service users receive from family carers, but only *after* a carers' assessment has been conducted, so that the service user's PB reflects the carer's *actual* willingness and ability to provide support. Transparent and equitable approaches to allocating resources to support carers in their own right are recommended, with maximum choice and control for carers over how those resources are used. Support plans should address the needs of both service users and carers, with services and support to sustain the caring role (as far as the carer wishes) included in the PB of the service user. This guidance can be seen as an attempt to graft local authorities' statutory responsibilities to carers onto personalisation processes. However, it does not address some important underlying issues and leaves many questions unanswered. For example, whose needs should be taken into account? Who should resources be directed at? To what extent should carers and service users be treated as separate individual units? What is the best way to optimise outcomes for both?

As increasing numbers of disabled and older people receive social care support in the form of PBs, it is important to examine how far carer and service user support processes are integrated or aligned, and how any tensions are acknowledged and managed in routine social care practice. This was the aim of the study described here. For brevity, throughout this chapter the term 'personalisation processes' is used to refer to processes of assessment, determining resource allocation, planning support, and ongoing management and review of support arrangements.

The study

The Carers and Personalisation study (2011–13) explored how far adult social care practice recognised and balanced the needs and wishes of service users and their carers.

The study involved the following:

- A survey of local policy/practice in two English regions (16 out of 29 councils completed the survey).
- In-depth investigation of practice in three of these 16 councils, through interviews with senior personalisation and carer lead managers (a total of six interviews) and nine focus groups (a total of 47 staff) involving qualified social workers and non-professional social care staff who conducted assessments from older people and learning disability teams.
- Individual interviews with carers and older and disabled people with cognitive or communication disabilities (14 carer and service user dyads).

The study focused on older and disabled people with cognitive or communication impairments, as their carers were likely to be heavily involved in personalisation processes. Findings can also be found in Brooks et al (forthcoming) and Mitchell et al (2014).

Carer involvement in service user assessment

In this study, staff recognised the inappropriateness of focusing solely on service users' needs and aspirations, and staff reported that carers of service users with cognitive or communication impairments were routinely involved in service user assessments. Carers and service users also emphasised the importance of carer involvement. Staff in learning disability teams felt they worked particularly closely with carers due to long-standing relationships with service users and their families. Carers themselves wanted to be involved, especially in social worker assessments, so they could help service users understand questions and contribute detailed information.

> 'I think my role's just to make sure that, you know [son's name] sort of giving a reasonable rendition of what they're asking him.... I mean I'm there if he gets something slightly wrong or can't remember.' (Carer of son with learning disabilities)

The majority of service users were happy about their carer's participation; few spoke to practitioners on their own, as they found talking to practitioners difficult.

> 'She [Mum] helped me with some questions....' (Service user with learning disabilities)

> '... someone was there who understood me.' (Older person service user)

Assessing carers' own needs

The role assigned to carers during personalisation depends on practitioners' perceptions, for example, as Twigg and Atkin (1994) suggest, a support resource or a co-client with their own support needs. Focusing on carers as a resource, local authorities have duties, as part of service user assessments, to ask carers about the support they give and their willingness and ability to continue providing this (DH, 2010e). In response to prompts on service user assessment forms, managers and staff confirmed that carers were routinely asked during service user assessments about their willingness and ability to continue caring and about any support they needed to do so. However, staff also reported using these prompts to ask carers about their own support needs, reflecting more of a co-client role. Some practitioners described these questions as 'mini' carer assessments nestled within service user assessments; others saw them as part of a 'joint' assessment. However, other practitioners regarded carer questions within service user assessments as too narrow, overlooking the emotional impact of caring.

> 'I think in a joint assessment you get the more practical things of what the carer does, I don't think you get so much about the emotional impact because I don't think they feel about to say that in front of their mother/father.' (Care practitioner)

Service user assessment forms also had limited space to record carers' needs and this was an issue of concern for some practitioners. Assessment forms designed around tick boxes did not allow detailed recording of carers support needs.

> '... the form pushes you more into thinking about how much the carer is doing rather than the impact it's having

on the carer. And I think if you haven't always considered the carer, I don't think that form necessarily says you're to do that, not really.' (Social worker)

Most carers recalled being asked whether they were willing and able to continue providing support, but could not remember being asked in detail about their own support needs, that is, as a co-client during service user assessments.

Reflecting the view of carers as co-clients (Twigg and Atkin, 1994), local authorities also have duties to inform carers of their right to a separate assessment of their own needs. Managers and staff reported that they informed carers of their rights to separate assessments, but beyond this there was little consistency and separate assessments of carers' support needs were far less common. Some practitioners were aware of the benefits of separate assessments for carers, acknowledging that they provided an opportunity for carers to discuss their own needs and the impact of caring in private. Some separate carer assessments were reported, but the timing of these varied and they could be conducted some time after the service user's assessment. There was also little agreement between managers and practitioners over whether the same practitioner should do both service user and carer assessments. Managers and staff reported that not all carers wanted a separate assessment, particularly if they had already contributed to the service user's assessment.

Having a separate assessment was recalled by some carers but not all could remember being offered one and others had declined the offer of a separate assessment because its relevance and purpose was unclear to them. Those carers who had had separate assessments valued opportunities to discuss the emotional aspects of caring with practitioners.

> 'She [social worker] came to the house, she had a nice cup of tea and she did have a bit of a checklist but was more a really good informal chat ... and it was nice 'cos it was actually how that affects you.' (Carer of son with learning disabilities)

However, such opportunities were reported as rare.

Carers and resource allocation

Practitioners reported that service users' PBs were reduced to reflect help given by carers, but there was little consistency or transparency in exactly how this was implemented. Most importantly, even when separate carer assessments were conducted, these were rarely linked to service user assessments so it was unclear how carers' own views about providing care, its impact and their own support needs would inform the level of the service user's PB.

Furthermore, practitioners' awareness of resources to support carers themselves was limited. Support for carers tended to be in the form of short breaks and these were commonly included within service users' PBs.

> '... almost always a good package of care and a good assessment of the service user does everything that the carer wants.' (Social worker)

Very few carers were reported to receive PBs of their own, although occasional one-off payments to carers (for example, for a washing machine) were reported by practitioners. These were usually funded and delivered separately, directly to carers themselves. How to allocate support to carers was a topic of ongoing debate for managers, as they had mixed views about developing separate resource allocation systems for carers. This fragmentation of resources between service user and carer budgets proved difficult for carers to understand.

Support planning

Practice guidance recommends that support planning should be led by service users, with carer involvement, and conducted *after* calculating an indicative service user PB (DH, 2010e). Carer involvement in service user support planning is important because, as the IB evaluation (Glendinning et al, 2009) concluded, this could be an indicator of positive outcomes for carers. However, practitioners in this study reported that it was often common practice for support planning discussions to take place at the same time as service user assessments. Hence, there appeared little opportunity for any separate carer assessments to influence the level of service users' PBs or support plans. It was also unclear, given the infrequency of separate carer assessments, how any information from these separate assessments about changes in carer circumstances would be reflected in revisions to service user budgets and support plans. Despite these practice inconsistencies, staff still reported that carers participated in service user support planning because of their routine involvement in service user assessments and the opportunities this gave carers to discuss service users' support needs.

Reflecting the reported low frequency of separate carer assessments, it comes as little surprise that there was an absence of evidence of carers having their own support plans that included employment, training or leisure activities. Carers themselves had low expectations of receiving such support.

Issues and implications

Findings from the study demonstrate the constraints and pressures that routine social care practice faces in trying to balance and take account of the needs and wishes of carers during service user assessments. Taken together, routine practice generally did not:

- link information from service user and carer assessments;
- ensure information from separate carer assessments contributed to service user support planning;
- ensure separate carer assessments were conducted before service user PB levels were adjusted to take account of help from carers.

These issues reflect the everyday practice problems practitioners face. These are due to structural design problems within a system of personalisation that fails to adequately recognise the rights of carers. Moreover, the inclusion of resources for carers' short breaks within the PB of the person they support does not appear to optimise carers' opportunities for choice and control, because these resources are under the control of the service user. This does not give carers equal rights on a par to those they cared for. However, recognising that the lives of carers (especially family carers) and those they support are often interwoven and interdependent can mean that good support arrangements for service users may go some way to meeting the needs of carers.

How to overcome tensions created by the separation of legislation and practice guidance regarding service users and carers also remains unresolved. It is not clear how far this separation will be remedied by the Care Act 2014 in England which aims to clarify, for example, responsibilities and to give carers similar rights and entitlements to service users. By strengthening carers' rights, the Act may simply intensify the challenges frontline practitioners face. Yet, at the same time, the interdependence and personal preferences of older and disabled people and their carers cannot be overlooked. It is thus important to recognise this variability in relationships between service users and carers and how this may affect how carers prefer to be assessed and have their support needs met. Some carers, for example spouse carers, may prefer to be treated as a single 'whole family' unit, whereas others, such as an adult child and his/her parent may want to be assessed and have their support needs met independently of each other. Standardised practice may not always be the most appropriate way to meet carer and service user individual needs. Although clearly there are no easy answers, working towards better coordinated service user and carer assessments and support plans continues to be important.

Despite this, it also remains important to recognise that it may not be possible to resolve the tensions inherent in the policies and practice of personalisation when these are based on wider assumptions of individualised consumerism and overlook the realities (as identified by Arksey and Glendinning, 2007, and Mitchell, 2012) of the diverse social contexts within which people receive (and give) care and make choices about that care.

Acknowledgements

This chapter presents independent research commissioned by the National Institute for Health Research (NIHR) School for Social Care Research. The views expressed in this publication are those of the authors and not necessarily those of the NIHR School for Social Care Research or the Department of Health, NIHR or NHS.

EIGHT

Self-funders:
the road from perdition?

Melanie Henwood

Personalisation is, above all, 'about giving people choice and control over their lives', and ensuring that care and support responds to people's needs and wishes and enables them to 'lead active, independent and connected lives' (HM Government, 2012). A key element in enabling people to exercise choice and control is the personal budget, particularly when taken in the form of a direct payment. It might be assumed that having purchasing power automatically gives people choice and control; this is the way that most markets operate. However, research into the experiences of people who are self-funding and buying their own social care support indicates that, on the contrary, this is often an isolated and disadvantaged pathway in which people are ill equipped to make informed decisions (Hudson and Henwood, 2009; Henwood, 2011). Having money alone does not necessarily enable people to take control unless they also have access to appropriate information, advice and advocacy.

The situation of people who are self-funding has – until very recently – been largely absent from the discourse around social care. The changes that are envisaged by the Care Act (2014) should, for the first time (from 2016 onwards), mean that people who pay for their own care have an incentive to approach their council for assessment, and that the council also has new duties to ensure the provision of information and advice and to monitor the spending of self-funders through an individual care account. In effect, this should offer self-funders greater opportunities to share in the wider benefits of personalisation being promoted for people using publicly funded care and support. This chapter explores the implications of the changes that are envisaged and considers how far removed this is from the current experience of most self-funders.

Understanding self-funders

The term 'self-funders' is used in a range of ways in social care discussion and refers to a wide spectrum of circumstances. Hudson and Henwood (2009) highlighted a continuum of definitions in common usage including people:

- part-funded by the council but paying the balance themselves;
- who *could* be eligible for council funding but haven't applied for an assessment;
- using personal budgets;
- paying for and arranging their own care and support, which can range from a 'little bit of help' about the house to permanent residential or nursing home care.

In this chapter, the term is used primarily to refer to the last of these categories and is therefore concerned with people who fund their own care from income, savings and capital. Currently, national regulations on paying for residential care require people with savings above £23,250 to meet the costs of their care in full. The Care Act 2014 changes this threshold and raises it significantly to £118,000 (discussed in more detail later in the chapter).

It is estimated that nationally around 45% of residential care home places and almost 48% of nursing home places, together with 20% of home care, is privately funded (IPC, 2011). Such estimates are likely to be incomplete, particularly in respect of home care where it can be difficult to distinguish between private care and private domestic help, and where much of this support occurs through informal and grey economies rather than through formal contracts and transactions with agencies and staff. Until recently there was relatively little qualitative research on the experience of people who self-fund – how they access the system or make their particular choices. A study by the former Commission for Social Care Inspection (CSCI) found self-funders 'often disadvantaged and isolated', and 'rather than making active choices, many appear to end up in situations as a matter of chance' (CSCI, 2008, p xii). Further research undertaken for the Putting People First Consortium (Henwood, 2011) similarly found that 'in almost every situation it was evident that people had not made their choices in a deliberate and planned way' (p 64). Major life-changing decisions were often made in crisis situations and on the basis of little or no information or advice on navigating the complex world of care and support. Far from exercising choice and control, many people experienced a profound sense of powerlessness and uncertainty, and lacked meaningful choices.

Policy and reform

The development of policy on eligibility for adult social care under both the present government, and the previous Labour administration, has included expectations on councils towards people who fund their own care. Guidance issued in 1998 was clear that local councils had a legal duty to assess the needs of anyone who might have 'need of community care services'. Moreover:

> Even if someone may be able to pay the full cost of any services, or make their own arrangements independently, they should be advised about what type of care they require and informed about what services are available. (Department of Health, 1998, para 8)

The guidance issued on Fair Access to Care Services in 2002 similarly underlined that assessment of needs must precede assessment of ability to pay, and that eligibility should be understood within a broader context, with 'adequate signposting to alternative sources of support' (DH, 2002, para 18).

Revised guidance was issued in February 2010 emphasising the importance of prevention and early intervention within a context of universal services, strengthening communities and establishing a model of support 'in which all citizens can expect some level of support and those with the greatest needs can access additional help' (DH, 2010c). This is often referred to as the concept of the 'universal offer' – the idea that everyone should have a right to assessment and information and advice.

Supporting better outcomes for everyone put particular emphasis on information and advice about other sources of support, as well as 'signposting to more universal sources of support'. Universal and open-access services have a particular role to play in helping people whose needs may be below eligibility thresholds, but where some early intervention can prevent or delay the need for care.

The government's *Vision for adult social care*, published in late 2010, underlined the same themes by identifying personalisation as one of seven principles for reform, and ensuring that 'information about care and support is available for all local people, regardless of whether or not they fund their own care' (DH, 2010a).

These issues were subsequently reinforced by the report of the Dilnot Commission on Funding of Care and Support in July 2011, with the recommendation that information and advice must be a universal service 'available to all, including those fully funding their own care' (Dilnot Commission, 2011, p 43). This was similarly a key recommendation of the Law Commission's proposals for reform of adult social care (Law Commission, 2011).

The White Paper *Caring for our future* (HM Government, 2012), published a year after the Dilnot report, expanded the vision and provided the basis for the Care Act (2014), establishing new duties around the promotion of wellbeing and independence, and the provision of information and advice to put people in control and enable them to plan ahead.

Despite the apparent intention of guidance and policy over several years that self-funders should not simply be left to find their own way, it is evident that in reality this is often the case. Work undertaken for CSCI in 2008 found that councils have historically adopted a continuum of positions towards people who fund their own care, ranging from a denial of any help, to minimalist information, and only a minority having a developed strategy in this area (CSCI, 2008b). Indeed, the experience of self-funders reflects some wider shortcomings in the approach of local councils to public information, advice and advocacy. Work commissioned by the Transforming Adult Social Care Programme Board in 2009 indicated that most local authorities had concentrated initially on 'developing the mechanisms and culture for personal budgets', while strategic approaches to information had been relatively neglected (Williams et al, 2009). As noted earlier, more recent research into the experience of self-funders has revealed the frequently poor experiences people have in trying to find out what support might be available to them, particularly if they have been turned away from social services as ineligible, or they fail to approach the council for help (Henwood, 2011). If people are screened out of assessment processes too soon because they are identified as self-funding, or they are given inadequate signposting to other sources of help, there are significant risks that prevention and reablement opportunities are lost, and that people are admitted prematurely to permanent residential care. The isolation and uncertainty about what to do were vividly described by research participants as these two carers of relatives paying for care illustrate:

> 'They just said "oh, she's self-funding" that was it, you know (...) somebody did come out from social services. She came

out to see Mother and to make an assessment. We never heard anything more.' (p 74)

'Here I was in a completely unknown and new situation as far as I was concerned, so I had got no idea what steps I should be taking with local authorities or social services or anybody. I hadn't got a clue.'(p 76)

Some people described the difficulties they experienced in trying to choose a care home for a relative and feeling uninformed in making the decision, with no opportunity to discuss options with someone who had the necessary expertise, rather than being passed from 'pillar to post'.

The Care Act and the Care Account

The reforms to be introduced through the Care Act 2014 are substantial and are a response both to the Dilnot Commission on funding, and the review of adult social care law by the Law Commission. For people who are funding their own care, there are some significant changes, in the Act:

- Local authorities 'must establish and maintain a service for providing people in its area with information and advice relating to care and support for adults and support for carers'.
- In addition to information about how to access care and support, information and advice must also be provided on how to access independent financial advice.
- Where a person has been assessed as having eligible needs but the local authority will not meet them because of the person's financial assets, the local authority must prepare an 'independent personal budget' that specifies what the cost would be to the local authority of meeting the person's eligible needs for care and support (that is, the 'notional cost' of meeting the adult's needs).
- The local authority must then keep an up to date record of the adult's accrued costs (a 'care account') and inform the person when the costs exceed the cap on care costs that they are required to pay themselves.

The lifetime contribution that people must make to their care has been set at £72,000 (and will be uprated in line with average earnings), and at the same time the means–testing upper capital threshold for residential care is to be raised from the present £23,250 to £118,000, and to £27,000 for non–residential care.

On the face of it, there will – for the first time – be positive reasons for people who believe they will be self-funding to approach their council for an assessment of their needs for care and support. Not only should there be improved access to information and advice (and vitally, independent financial advice), but the cost of meeting eligible needs will be monitored and people will not face potentially unlimited liability and catastrophic care costs. This would seem to be an improvement on the current situation when self-funders can spend below the means-testing threshold with no knowledge or awareness of what help they might be entitled to, and where local authorities may be unaware of the existence of self-funders until care home residents run out of money.

However, the care account will not monitor the amount that people *actually* spend on their care, but the amount that the local authority *would expect to pay*. The difference could be significant; this is not just because people might 'choose' to buy more expensive care, but also because it reflects the reality that self-funders typically are charged higher rates in residential care than local authorities are able to negotiate, and effectively self-funders subsidise publicly funded places. Moreover, the cap applies only to the 'care' element of costs and not the 'hotel' component of residential care. Commentators have pointed out that in practice people will therefore pay out considerably more than the capped cost by the time they reach the cap (and the costs of support to meet low or moderate needs will not be metered at all or count towards the care cap because it will be below the eligibility threshold). Moreover, in reality most people needing care and paying for it themselves will *never* reach the cap. People will also see their care account progressing at very different rates according to where they live and the usual rate that councils pay for care. Some analysis has suggested that this could vary between an average of three years' residential care to eight years depending on location (Lloyd, 2013). There will also be significant implementation costs associated with these reforms, not least as a consequence of the additional numbers of people who will present themselves for an assessment of their needs (and means), and in the subsequent administration of care accounts.

Some of the claims that the government has made for the capped cost model may not be experienced by people in practice. In particular, the model has been promoted as offering greater fairness and certainty to the public. However, if, as Lloyd argues, the 'capped cost' does not in practice cap what people have to pay, and the new upper capital limit does not result in people getting financial help that they expect, there could be a loss of confidence in the reformed system and considerable confusion (Lloyd, 2013).

People will need to have confidence in the existence and operation of a care cap if they are to see any benefit in having contact with their local authority. Certainly, the availability of better information and advice on making contact could be an incentive, and being able to make choices and informed decisions about the options available could be significantly different from the current situation. The policy statement issued by the Department of Health in February 2013 stated that providing information and advice for self-funders 'in turn will make care services more responsive and more personalised, helping to drive up quality and create a more diverse care market'(DH, 2013b, para 29).

The vital role of information and advice, and the need for local authorities to be proactive in providing this, has been highlighted during the passage of the Care Act 2014 through parliament. Indeed, at a very late stage of the journey, in the third reading in the House of Lords, discussions took place about the need for regulations and guidance to ensure that councils take a 'facilitative role' and provide self-funders with 'a nudge in an appropriate direction' towards independent, regulated financial advice. Earl Howe – among others – argued that 'handing out a leaflet or placing a page on a website is not sufficient' (House of Lords, 2013). The significance of the response that needs to be put in place is underlined by findings in 2011 that only 3% of councils were signposting people to independent financial advisors who could give advice about care funding products (Carr-West and Thraves, 2011).

Assessment will be at the heart of the reformed system, and this will be located within a new national eligibility framework. The argument is that rather than simply acting as a gateway to a person either receiving care and support or not,

> the future system will place more emphasis on the role of the assessment process in supporting people to identify their needs, understand the options available to them, plan for meeting care needs and for caring responsibilities and reduce or delay needs where possible. (DH, 2013c, para 1.8)

The magnitude of the cultural shift in the role of councils, social workers and care assessors will be substantial, as several reports have acknowledged. For example, work on the principles that should underpin the provision of information and advice published by the Think Local, Act Personal partnership (TLAP, 2013b) emphasises that 'good information is at the heart of good decision-making, and it enables people to maintain control over their lives'. Councils will 'need to develop a culture of information-sharing and an information and advice strategy' that encompasses multiple dimensions. An 'interactive map' developed to highlight the 'pinch points' where councils need to pay particular attention in improving the information and advice offer to people and their families similarly indicates the enormity of the transformation required (Bottery and Holloway, 2013).

A guide for health and wellbeing boards and commissioners published by the Office for Public Management has sketched out the challenges to be addressed with the transition to a new funding system, and stated that 'there is a strong argument that commissioners should treat self-funding as another type of self-directed support, and aim to enable a social care market that works well for all' (Miller et al, 2013, p 5).

Nonetheless, all of these new responsibilities towards self-funders will take place at a time of growing financial pressure on local authorities, in which – according to the Association of Directors of Adult Social Services – a bleak outlook is getting bleaker. Between 2011-12 and 2013-14, adult services departments have had to find savings of 20% net spending (ADASS, 2013a). Service efficiencies have been achieved but it is now recognised that reductions in service will increasingly be required to achieve further savings, and this will create significant tensions with the new role and responsibilities envisaged for local councils in the Care Act.

Conclusion

The experiences of people who are funding their own care and support are diverse, but most people do not find that simply having some purchasing power enables them to make real choices or to get the support that is best suited to their needs. The reforms to adult social care that are to take effect from 2016 have the *potential* to change this situation substantially, to improve access to independent information and advice, and to create positive reasons for people to seek assessment of their needs from adult social care departments. This would be a major step forward, but whether such benefits will be achieved will reflect many variables.

For local councils the challenge will be profound in moving from a model that has often been seen as gatekeeping and protecting demands on public money, to one that supports people to maintain their independence and achieve their objectives and preferences. The training implications alone will be significant if the system is no longer to see it as appropriate for inquiry into assets and savings to be the first question a person is asked when they seek help. Similarly, information and advice will need to become far more active and dynamic, and 'signposting' must no longer be a euphemism – as is often the reality – for 'no help available here'. There will also be challenges in developing the provider market, both in securing information, advice and brokerage services, as well as in stimulating care and support providers to recognise the need to respond to the self-funder market.

Above all, people paying for care will need confidence in, and clear understanding of, the new system. Given the confusion that currently surrounds adult social care, and the poor experiences of many self-funders in seeking help, the scale of the transformation required to ensure personalised support for all cannot be overstated.

Part Three
Frontline perspectives

NINE

Managing direct payments

Christine Bond

In this chapter, I outline my personal experiences and views of using a personal budget and managing direct payments (DPs). I have received support packages both under the old assessment process and have had a personal budget for over four years, all of which have had some form of a DP element. Having social care needs is not a choice. It was not until I reached crisis point and came to terms with my situation that I asked for help and started to receive a personal care package. To me, having a personal budget is more than just money, as no amount of money is going to resolve all of the challenges and barriers I face on a day-to-day basis; it is about giving me the resources and enabling me to decide how to manage my life and conditions to the best of my ability through more tailored and flexible support. After all, who has exactly the same needs even if they have the same conditions?

The journey

After meeting the eligibility and financial criteria, I completed a personal budget questionnaire, which covers the different tasks I carry out in my life, both practical and emotional. I answered the questions as if I had no support, including unpaid care, and was then asked (along with the unpaid carer) how much unpaid support they were prepared to give and what support they needed to do this. An indicative budget was calculated based on the answers (jointly agreed by myself and my allocated worker) to the questions posed.

Once I had an amount, the next stage was to write a support plan. As well as explaining how my budget was going to be spent and managed, it also covered what was important to me, what was working well and not, my desired goals/outcomes and how I planned to keep myself safe. It wasn't until I had a personal budget that I was asked about the more positive side of my situation. Writing this document was the key process to helping me to work out how my needs were going to be met and managed based on my support/care needs (as identified in the questionnaire).

The plan is my plan, written by me with the support of others if I choose. It still has to be approved by a professional to make sure I have covered all my needs and that I stay safe, but the power to decide how this is achieved has moved towards me rather than a professional and it is at this point that the final budget is agreed. Going through this process each year has helped me to continually shape support plans to reflect the changes in my life, including what will happen if things go wrong in the short term (my contingency plan). Having a 'contingency plan' was something new to me and having one in place gives me the reassurance of what to do in an emergency (for example, what I will do if my main family carer is unable to provide the support I need due to illness or other unforeseen circumstances). If my needs change in the long term (like under the old system), I know that I can contact community (social) services and have my needs reassessed.

When thinking about how to manage my budget, I can choose between community services or another third party holding my money on my behalf, having a DP or a combination. There is no right or wrong answer, but each decision will have its benefits and disadvantages. I have found that passing the responsibility to someone else costs a bit more due to the extra administration involved and is less flexible. Having a DP gives me more control, but I am responsible for making sure that payments are being made and that I have enough money to pay them. Where I live there is an agency that can help me manage my budget. Having a DP does not necessarily mean that I have to employ my own support as it may be used for things like agency care, breaks away, respite care, equipment or attending a day service, centre or activity.

Having a personal budget has given me the freedom to think differently. To start with my care package was very similar to what I received before, as it included personal care (DPs to employ my own staff and/or use agencies), supported activities and breaks away/respite care. However, as I identified what was not working so well, I was able to alter how I received my support to better meet my circumstances. I know of several different people who have been more creative with their packages, but for me the most important things I needed was personal assistant (PA) support and for my husband to have a break. This was particularly important as I was unable to use other finances to pay for any extra care I needed through the current system. Even though on paper the old and new care packages look similar, one of the biggest differences has been flexibility of my chosen care arrangements and having a back-up plan if things go wrong. The new system looked at what could go wrong, how this could be prevented and if not what action should take place. I have also found that completing a questionnaire makes sure that all aspects of my support needs are taken into account rather than just those that tend to come up in conversation. Although the questionnaires have been refined over the years, this process has also has given me some idea/comparison of how my needs have changed over the year. Overall, I have found the whole process has been more flexible and with a greater opportunity of deciding how my care needs are met.

In addition to having a personal budget, I receive additional funding for equipment and to employ a support worker from Jobcentre Plus through a government scheme called Access to Work (ATW). This scheme provides grants for people with a disability, health or mental health condition to either go into or stay in employment. This funding provides the tailored support I need to carry out my work duties. For example, as I am no longer able to drive and my work involves going to several different locations, I can employ a support worker to drive me to wherever I need to go. More information about the ATW scheme can be found on the gov.uk website (www.gov.uk/access-to-work/overview). This funding has enabled me to stay in employment for many years but there is limited support available to help with the complicated processes of accessing and using the scheme.

In Norfolk I was part of a personal health budget pre-pilot, which involved developing a health plan template and trialling the process of a health budget. I then completed the support plan with the help of a key worker. The plan was used to explain my preferences, goals and how I planned to spend the budget to meet my particular needs. Like the personal budget plan, it was my plan, and I chose which sections I wanted to complete, including adding any supporting documents. Again this made me think differently, giving me more power and confidence to shape the direction I wanted my health needs to go in (not all of which had a financial cost). At this stage, no specific funds were allocated as it was a pilot with the aim of seeing what people would ask for and testing how the system might work but it had to be approved by a panel. Funding criteria were later developed for the main pilot. At this point I requested a mixture of alternative therapies (which I could have at home) that would help to either reduce the amount of medication I was on or at least stop it from increasing. To start with, the therapists were paid directly and when the law was changed I received a direct payment. The whole process was monitored regularly. The funding and the health plan have made a real difference and having all my medical information I wanted in one place has helped a lot with communication and explaining my situation to health professionals and community services. This is a completely new way of working and most health professionals have taken my wishes on board, although not everyone has understood the importance of my health plan. This has worked alongside my PB support plan but it would be better if the two documents could in some way be amalgamated. I have had a personal health budget for a total of three years, but the pilot has come to an end and future funding at present is uncertain because of the decision to fund personal health budgets only for people on Continuing Healthcare. However, I have had the support of my GP and specialist and we are now looking at how my alternative therapies can be funded in the future.

The advantages of a personal budget

One of the key benefits of having a personal budget for me has been the flexibility of my care package. Having a condition that can be so varied and can change very quickly has always been difficult to manage. This was one of the biggest problems under the old DP system, as the number of hours of support I received each week tended to be fixed and, if they were not used within eight weeks, the money was taken back (which was known as 'the eight-week rule'). On the other hand, with my personal budget, I have been allocated an amount of money for my whole care package for a 12-month period. This amount has been worked out on the number of hours of support I think I might need during the year at an agency rate per hour, but it can also be used to employ my own staff. This means that I have the option of using my own PAs, which I prefer, but if they are not available for any reason, I know that I have a fixed number of agency hours within a year that I can draw on. Having my needs assessed on a yearly basis (although this can be stressful) allows me to re-evaluate my support package and ensures that I am receiving the right support for my needs. I have a similar arrangement regarding using my own PAs for my morning care, as agencies have not been as flexible as I have needed them to be.

Finding suitable PAs has also been a challenge both under the old and new systems, especially when living in a rural area, as I only have funding for a few hours per week, and the times when I need care are fragmented over the day. This challenge has been made easier with a personal budget because it allows me some flexibility with the hourly rate I can pay my staff. However, as there is no extra money to increase the hourly rate it is important to find the right balance between the number of hours you want and the hourly rate you can pay.

The issues and how they have been resolved

To obtain the flexibility I need in my life I have had to become an employer, which is a big responsibility and is not something I would have chosen if it were not for my personal care needs. It is important that my PAs are paid and treated correctly and that all the necessary legislation, including health and safety requirements, are adhered to. This includes making sure that my staff have the adequate training for the tasks I am expecting them to perform in order to prevent them from injuring themselves or me. Some of this training I have done myself, as it is very specific to my condition, but I have been lucky enough to access some free training through community services. Some additional money was set aside in my budget to cover any future training needs.

Working out accurate employment costs has been one of the hardest things, as it is not just a matter of working out how much to pay your staff per hour; you need also to take into account all the on-costs, like employers' National Insurance, bank holiday pay, holiday entitlement, sick pay and maternity/paternity pay. I have chosen to use an organisation that has been commissioned by my local authority to provide support to people who are employing their own staff. Support includes helping to recruit new staff, writing employment contracts, providing advice on employment issues/law, accounting services, including making payments, running payroll and completing the monitoring requirements of the council and HM Revenue & Customs.

What needs to be done to make personal budgets work well?

The introduction of personal budgets has, and will continue to bring, new challenges. Everyone has to think differently. Individuals with care needs will have the opportunity to tailor the way they receive support to meet their needs; service providers need to think about individual wants as well as needs, and how they can remain viable in this new environment; and statutory authorities need to ensure that their staff, policies and procedures are flexible enough to ensure that individuals have true flexibility and choice in their support packages. For things to work well, new ways of working will have to be created rather than trying to bolt on to existing ways of doing things. It is also important that there is no gap between one budget ending and the next one starting.

In the past few years, I have seen my package go from a very rigid and structured package to a very flexible and responsive budget. I know what my needs are, but the best way to meet them has been a challenge and that is why information and support (both at the start of the process and during it) has been so important. This can be provided in many different ways and what works for one person might be unsuitable for another, so it is important that there are different ways this can be provided that are accurate and up to date. One of the best ways for me was having the opportunity to talk to other people with care needs, both people who fund their own care as well as those receiving social care (peer support). I have been lucky, as I have a good peer support network coordinated by a county-wide, user-led organisation and funded by the county council. Peer support is not just about face-to-face meetings but could also be achieved through online forums or by setting up Skype groups. Having good peer support groups, no matter what form they may take, can be a good opportunity for local councils and providers to talk to people and find out what can be done to improve their services. Having a collective voice not only helps to obtain more views but also helps those who are less willing or able to express themselves individually. As well as being a way of sharing information/experiences, it could also help people to share their resources (collective purchasing). In times of austerity, this could allow individuals to make better use of the money allocated with the potential of opening up more opportunities. Collective purchasing should not just be for those on PBs, but should also involve individuals with other funding streams so that even greater opportunities are available.

If individuals are going to have true choice and control, it is important that there are providers in place that can help individuals (especially those who wish to employ their own PAs) by providing help with support planning, employment support, a payroll service and supported accounts, as this will help to create a more level playing field for everyone no matter what their needs are. Professionals who are supporting individuals with their personal budgets need to have a good overall understanding of the whole process, as everything is connected and any one element will have an impact on other parts of the care package. Ideally, there should be a choice of providers who are able to cover people with a variety of needs so that providers do not just pick those with the easier care packages to manage. If there is more than one organisation or department involved in providing a person's support, there needs to be good communication (with the individual's permission) to ensure the smooth running of the budget.

If the local authority decides to change DPs annually, it is important that the new amounts are clearly explained and, if recipients are employing their own staff, that there is support to work out the new rates and what impact these will have, especially if an individual's budget starts at a different time of the year.

It is my hope that eventually there will be one budget/funding stream with one set of rules that will cover all my support and care needs. I could not achieve what I have done in my life without support, but having to rely on different funding steams has also caused a lot of problems and unnecessary stress, as some payments are paid four weeks in advance (DPs) and others only available after the hours have been worked (ATW). All my costs have been split between my PB and ATW and I spend a lot of time filling in the necessary paperwork, timesheets and monitoring of both funding streams. I also have to go through several different assessments, which are reviewed at different times.

To summarise, personal budgets for me are a good thing, as I have more flexibility, choice and control over managing my requirements. How you decide to manage your budget should be down to your personal preference and not the amount of support available from both professionals and peers. The systems in place offered by providers and local authorities should be easy to use with the minimum amount of paperwork and flexible enough (including collective purchasing and joint funding streams) to meet the needs of the people who use them. Professionals and others working with people with care needs should have a good understanding of the whole process so that they can provide better support to the people they work with. Lastly, this way of working is still bringing new challenges and everyone has to think differently for things to work well.

TEN

Beyond 'being an employer': developing micro-markets

Sian Lockwood

The government strategy to drive personalisation focused in the early days almost entirely on giving people personal budgets (then called individual budgets). Targets were set for the percentage of people with a personal budget and the assumption was that giving people the money would drive the development of new types of supports and services and deliver personalisation:

> Giving people an individual budget should drive up the quality of services. The ability of people to 'buy' elements of their care or support package will stimulate the social care market to provide the services people actually want, and help shift resources away from services which do not meet needs and expectations. We intend that the introduction of individual budgets will help promote the more effective use of the resources available to meet care needs. (DH, 2005, p 34)

The money provided by government to local authorities to implement personalisation was principally used to develop complex resource allocation systems to decide the size of each person's personal budget. Local authorities had a responsibility for market shaping – ensuring that people had choice of services to buy with their budget – but, as with central government, broadly assumed that the mere fact that they were giving people money to buy their own support would drive the development of new services – and that anyway people would, and should, principally use their personal budget to directly employ their own staff.

Since the early days of the In Control individual budgets pilots, evidence has gathered of the positive impact of personal budgets on people's lives – but also that this impact is dependent on people being genuinely in control of the way the money is spent, having good information and real choice of a range of good local services. For most local authorities, giving people real control, comprehensive and accessible information and real choice is proving even more difficult than giving them a personal budget. 'There is a widespread perception that "real" personalisation means supported direct payments, with the person having to act as employer and co-ordinator of their support' (Hatton, 2013).

But not everyone wants to become an employer, especially not if their budget is too small for this to be a meaningful way of getting support; they lack the capacity to understand the issues and do not have a circle of people around them who can help; the right people are not available for them to employ; they find the responsibility of becoming an employer burdensome and are concerned about what happens if their personal assistant (PA) is sick or goes on holiday; or the approach has gone wrong in the past.

> Twitter provides revealing 'real-time' commentary on the limitations and difficulties of using personal budgets when there is little choice apart from the choice to become an employer:
>
> '... really, how is the only choice between **** home care services and being an employer.'
>
> 'I love having a PA. But seriously, whoever thought up the idea of "being an employer" to get direct payments needs spanking!'
>
> 'I need to set up payroll services, insurance and contracts and meet my advocate re DASS complaint. This really isn't an easy way to get support.'

A narrow focus on direct payments as a vehicle that allows people to employ their own support is one of the reasons for the flat-lining in the take-up of direct payments by people offered a personal budget. If there were real choice of good local support and services, people were helped to think creatively and imaginatively about the ways in which they could spend their money and had really good information about the options open to them, direct payments would become a really attractive option for more people.

Community Catalysts (www.communitycatalysts.co.uk) is a Community Interest Company working through local partners such as councils and third sector infrastructure organisations to help local people use their gifts, talents and imagination to set up sustainable social care and health enterprises. At Community Catalysts, we have a particular take on this subject, informed by our experiences of working through local partners to help people in communities use their gifts and skills to provide real choice of small-scale, local, personalised and high-quality social care and health services (in the broadest sense) for other local people looking for support and services. Our 'micro-entrepreneurs' may use services themselves, care for a loved one or have previously worked in social care. Some have no previous social care experience but have a passion or an interest that they want to introduce to people in their community – some of whom happen to have some support needs. Services may be delivered on a voluntary basis, as part of a cooperative or as a small social enterprise or business. In all cases, because of their size they are highly individualised, flexible and responsive. The examples below illustrate the variety and flexibility of these small community enterprises.

Companions is a small enterprise operating in a rural part of Oldham and founded by Susan Shaw, who has varied experience of supporting older people. Companions 'aims to be there for older people when friends and family can't'. The inspiration to run an independent service was born out of frustration that as a care worker certain tasks were laid out in a person's care plan and Sue had to stick to those tasks. Care was often rushed and impersonal when what people really wanted was a chat!

Staff at Companions are matched to customers as much as possible and change is kept to a minimum. Remaining small has enabled Sue to stick to her values of providing a person-centred service – one where the customer really feels like they care! Companions offers reassurance and help with everyday activities both inside and outside the home. Customers and families value the support provided as the excerpt from this letter from a family member shows: 'Thank you very much for your service and consideration you gave my mother in helping her to keep in her home for as long as possible. Nothing was too much trouble for your staff in taking her out on Saturdays and trying to keep her life normal.'

This year Sue was invited to attend the Queen's Garden Party in recognition of her great work in supporting local people in their community.

Ace of Spades was set up by Dave and Sarah, who live and work in the East Midlands, have a passion for gardening and have skills and experience in delivering care services. The service offers older people (particularly people with dementia) an opportunity to garden at a pace and level that they feel comfortable with. It encourages their physical and psychological well-being by providing opportunities to work outdoors, enjoy the natural environment and maintain what may have been a lifelong hobby or interest. Ace of Spades is especially enjoyed by older people who used to love gardening and people caring for an older family member who want to maintain their garden and enable the person they care for to take part in an activity that they used to enjoy.

Our work is both inspiring and frustrating. We are continually delighted by the passion, imagination and commitment of our community entrepreneurs, but, like them, can become frustrated by the many barriers placed in the way. We know that people with control of their own money and good information choose services and support that enable them to live their life – and that, in this environment, local community enterprise flourishes. In practice, we find, however, that control is mainly exercised by people with direct payments or people funding their own support, as those with managed budgets face limitations on choice that prevent them from buying local small-scale, non-traditional services.

Councils often inadvertently place barriers in the way of people with managed budgets exercising real choice – and in the process severely limit local market diversity. For example, councils may say that people with managed budgets can only buy services from providers on an approved list or framework contract. Getting a place on an approved list can be almost impossible for very small services offering something out of the ordinary and with very limited resources. Requirements are often inappropriate for very small services, as the case study below demonstrates:

Blossom Forth was set up by two single mums with disabled children to provide help in the home for other people in the same position. They knew at first hand how stressful it can be to care for a disabled child and wanted to use the skills and knowledge that they had gained from caring for their own children to help other families. They wanted to be able to offer direct care to the disabled child to free parents to spend time with their other children – or simply to have a break – and so applied to register with the Care Quality Commission as a domiciliary care agency. This process was tricky enough for a very small organisation run by people who had no formal educational qualifications but with a wealth of life experience. The real barrier came though when they tried to widen their offer to people using local authority-commissioned services and applied to be accepted onto the council's approved list. Domiciliary care agencies who wanted acceptance onto the approved list had to install an electronic call monitoring system and this requirement could not be varied just because the agency supported a very

> small number of clients (just eight families and with a planned maximum of 15). The cost was significant but perhaps more importantly the partners felt that the system skewed their working practices and damaged their ability to deliver good outcomes for people.

This type of limitation is usually the result of a local interpretation of European Union procurement rules. There are other restrictions imposed because of the need to control spending that both limit choice and have perverse and unanticipated impacts. An example is where the local authority caps the daily rate that can be paid for a day service. This obviously prevents the individual from choosing a more expensive service, perhaps balancing that with a service that costs less or is provided on a voluntary basis. It also damages the gift element contained within many community enterprises. The majority of micro-enterprises operate within what the International Futures Forum (2011) calls the 'gift economy'. Many of them of course receive payment for their work but while money is a motivator (we all need to eat), the key drivers are about connecting to other people, giving to the community they live in, valuing other people and feeling valued in return. The services they provide are grounded in relationships and in giving and receiving from each other. A set daily rate that does not take account of the cost to them of delivering their service (and that by implication does not value the service they are delivering) disheartens current micro-providers and perversely discourages all but the most commercial community entrepreneurs from establishing new day services.

There is a more subtle limitation on choice experienced by both people with managed budgets and people with direct payments, linked to the quality of the information about support options that is provided to budget holders. For example, a council may contract with an external support broker to help people with direct payments make good choices about how to spend their money. The support broker may specialise in helping people with direct payments to employ their own staff and may have very limited knowledge about the other kinds of supports and services available locally. Someone advised by such a broker, unless they are very determined, will be channelled into becoming an employer. Some councils keen to enable people with managed budgets to have more choice are creating individual services funds that are managed by external providers. Our experience, though, is that these providers, while not limited by EU procurement rules in the same way as local authorities, have limited knowledge of the support options available for people. Many local authorities see electronic directories as the way to fulfil their duty to provide accessible information to people with personal budgets. Each e-directory has its own access rules for providers wanting to advertise their service, and some of these are unintentionally biased to more traditional forms of provision. Local authorities keen to ensure that they provide information about the widest possible range of types of provider can struggle to identify and engage the very smallest provider. Many micro-enterprises operate under the radar of the local authority and it takes dedicated time, experience and skill to identify and engage with them.

The severe squeeze on public sector finances is leading to other practices that are reducing market diversity and therefore choice for people who need some support to lead the life they want to live. Many local authorities are considering 'spinning out' their direct care provision and in some areas they have done this wholesale, creating an arms-length organisation (ALMO) under council control to run their care services. This can in effect create a market monopoly where it is assumed that people with managed personal budgets will buy services from the ALMO. Information about other options will be given if people ask – but they need to know to ask.

The study carried out by York University's Social Policy Research Unit on personalisation and older people supports our empirical findings (Baxter et al, 2013). It found that older people tended to prefer council-managed personal budgets, but then had limited choice and control over their support:

> The biggest cause was the low value of managed budgets, which mostly only covered essential personal care, limiting the scope for money to be used flexibly once these needs had been met. However, this was exacerbated by commissioning practices that limited people's choice of provider and council restrictions over the way budgets were spent. While service users technically had a choice of providers on councils' framework agreements, often just one care agency was able to respond to a referral from a new client, with particular restrictions in rural areas. (Samuel, 2013b)

This catalogue of commissioning and contracting practices could lead you to conclude that the most positive personalised outcomes will always be experienced by people with direct payments employing their own support staff and that real market diversity is impossible to achieve in social care. Our experience, however, is that even in the most difficult financial times there are enlightened local authorities struggling to reform long-established commissioning and procurement practices and to find the money to stimulate and support micro-enterprise in order to ensure that people with personal budgets (managed or not) have real choice. And in these local authority areas community enterprise is thriving – creating not just choice for people but also new jobs and volunteering opportunities and delivering better value for money. Nottinghamshire County Council is one such authority.

Nottinghamshire County Council has made a four-year investment in local micro-enterprise. The project began in July 2010 and over that period:

- 240+ enquires have been received from members of the public in Nottinghamshire.
- 160 people have received active support and guidance from the support coordinator.
- 57 micro-enterprises are now operating across Nottinghamshire offering care and support services. These 57 micro-enterprises support over 860 people who need care and support to live their life. Between them they have created 112 jobs and 84 volunteering opportunities.
- 53 of these are new services established over the life of the project.
- There has been extensive regional and national recognition of the project.
- A large number of creative and innovative services are now available.
- Services are available to people in traditionally hard-to-reach groups or locations, including the rural north of the county.

There is work being done by Think Local, Act Personal and the Department of Health to try to encourage more imaginative commissioning and procurement practices, which will be helped when the European Union publishes its new 'light-touch' procurement rules (due to become law in the UK by the middle of 2014). This work will be helpful in liberating councils from practices that limit choice for people.

The challenge is that enlightened local authorities are in the minority. Enabling people to have real choice so that their personalised budgets become meaningful needs determination, focus and some resource – at a time when people in local authorities have ever-widening spans of responsibility and little resource. The financial challenges facing local authorities are significant and some, perhaps a significant number, are beginning to see real personalisation as a luxury that can no longer be afforded.

Furthermore there are some who think that the personalisation train has left the station. The hot topic at the National Children and Adult Care Services (England) conference 2013 was health and social care integration, which comes with significant funding from government (£2.7 billion plus an extra £100m in 2013/14 and a further £200 million in 2014/15). Making personalisation a reality is hard work. When the new money is all associated with integration, local authorities may be pardoned for taking their eye off the personalisation ball. Organisations like Community Catalysts working to help make personalisation a reality will need to work harder than ever to make sure that does not happen.

ELEVEN

What about the workforce?

Helga Pile

Personalisation in social care is a policy that started life with grand ambitions to 'transform' care and support. But there has been relatively little detailed discussion of role of the workforce in bringing about this transformation, and how it needs to change. This lack of emphasis on workforce has meant many councils have struggled to articulate a compelling workforce strategy. Little in the way of national policy leadership around this question has filtered down to the front line.

As personalisation began to roll out in local authorities, UNISON branches reported varying degrees of engagement with local employers around implementation. Some branches were able to secure very positive involvement. For example, a UNISON branch in the Midlands reported that it had negotiated to have a 'choice and control representative' working closely with the council, including sitting on the workforce project board and securing a learning partnership agreement. This kind of engagement helped with communicating and engaging with staff, winning their confidence and allowing them to have a say in the changes afoot.

However, in other areas there was little attempt to involve the unions, and for many staff the strategic vision behind personalisation is still proving slippery to grasp. Meanwhile, consultation with staff has tended to focus in on restructuring and changing processes. Frontline workers feel there was little attempt to convey the policy objectives behind personalisation. And for many the first tangible manifestations of personalisation have been negative in terms of them and their jobs. For example:

- Day centres have closed, jobs gone and the direct payments that have been put in their place are only enough to employ a personal assistant for a few hours a week (Needham, 2012).
- There is uncertainty about demand (direct payments uptake could lead to fewer users and therefore job losses).
- Councils have decided to outsource in-house services to arms-length companies or independent providers on the spurious grounds that

service users cannot use their direct payment to buy council services. They have not been willing to build on the strengths of in-house services to make them more flexible and responsive for users who do not opt for direct payments.
• Personalisation has triggered further substitution of lower graded posts for professionally qualified posts (discussed in more detail later).

Successive surveys (Community Care et al, 2010, 2011, 2012, 2013) of practitioners have highlighted growing concerns about bureaucracy associated with the new assessment processes. This letter from a UNISON branch to its local employer, copied to UNISON's head office, illustrates the frustrations and disempowerment that many have experienced:

> The introduction of self-directed support was predicated on the premise that individuals seeking social care services would be empowered to take control of a transparently open, objective and personalised assessment process that would flexibly accommodate their professed needs. In turn staff would also benefit by being able to practice in a manner that incorporates proactive and progressive social work values. In reality however budget constraints together with the need to ensure that all public expenditure is legitimately sanctioned has undermined these professed aims.

The branch went on to outline the issues that members were raising, including that:

• administrative demands have increased threefold;
• the fragmented and successive stages in the process are causing unreasonable delays;
• if the personal budget figure is higher than the current service provided, managers are indicating a need not to spend up to the allocated figure to safeguard the community care budget.

Role and skill mix

Because the process of support planning under personalisation is supposed to be led by the person with care and support needs, many local authorities have made the simple leap that they do not need to employ as many qualified social workers. This development was then seized upon by the Audit Commission and promoted as a simple means of reducing costs (Audit Commission, 2012a).

An informed and evidence-based national debate about skill mix in adult social work is long overdue. In the NHS, there are defined roles and learning and development pathways for assistant practitioners working alongside professional roles. But in social work these roles have developed entirely ad hoc – there are no nationally recognised training and development standards and no consistency in how paraprofessional staff are deployed, supervised and supported. The blurring of boundaries with professionally qualified roles creates the growing suspicion among practitioners that these changes are driven primarily by cost-cutting rather than optimising the skill mix (UNISON, 2011).

Many authorities have carried out restructuring of their adult social care teams linked to personalisation. This has split up functions along the care and support pathway: assessment is carried out by one team; support planning is then taken over by another. In some cases it is a third team – or a contracted out brokerage service – that works on facilitating access to the agreed services and support in place. And finally, a fourth team may be responsible for service reviews. For the service user this means multiple relationships and fragmentation. It also means complex record keeping and data input.

Practitioners working in one authority that had reorganised in this way commented to UNISON that "the assessment/care planning split is ridiculous and causes a great deal of inconsistency and confusion for the client", and that "the system where a professional worker assesses the customer and then passes the customer's case to a semi-professional to actually put services in is self-evidently a slower process than the same person assessing and then putting in services immediately or as soon as they are able".

There is also concern about what may be lost when assessment becomes a very time-limited process and there is no opportunity to refine or adjust to complexities, which may be identified through continuing work with the service user as the following extract from a UNISON report shows: 'The new system devalues the role of the skilled practitioner.... Brokers who are not trained social workers are more likely to miss the key dynamics' (UNISON, 2009, p 11). The report goes on:

> They should resist the temptation to replace social work posts with cheaper, unqualified staff. They should recognise that as the older population increases, so will the amount of complex, high risk work eg dementia, adult protection,

carer stress. Reductions in the qualified workforce now will eventually lead to more care disasters in future, and this damage to the skill level of the workforce will take years to undo. (UNISON, 2009, p 14)

From care assistants to personal assistants?

With the introduction of personalisation, pundits predicted a massive shift in the care delivery workforce away from staff working in the domiciliary care sector into a personal assistant workforce directly employed by service users, facilitating all aspects of their employers' lives including work, study, civic duties and leisure. Personal assistants were conceptualised as a greenfield workforce, separate from 'traditional' care workers, and more malleable. They would offer service users greater control because their employment could be entirely flexible. This would be in stark contrast to traditional care services where service users had to accept whoever was sent to them, at whatever time was convenient to the care agency, to perform only those tasks the professionals had decided could be done. So personalisation would focus on giving the user control by giving them power over the individual care worker. There was little exploration of alternatives that would have given them more power over the care agency, as this was hard to marry with the contracted-out care delivery model.

However, it is difficult to establish how far the shift to directly employed personal assistants has gone. Robust data on the personal assistant workforce is difficult to come by. The work done by Skills for Care, the employer-led workforce development body for social care in England, starts with the number of direct payment recipients in England and extrapolates figures for personal assistants (PAs) from there. This approach suggested there were 355,000 PA jobs employed by direct payment recipients in 2010 (Fenton, 2011). But the figure has now been revised downwards to 234,000 jobs following a methodology change to no longer treat all direct payment recipients as employers. These 234,000 workers are said to be employed by 100,000 direct payment recipients, which would mean an average of over two jobs per recipient (Skills for Care, 2013). This may still be an over-estimate.

From UNISON's work in this area, we know that many personal assistants in the UK combine multiple jobs, including jobs in formal social care settings or work for multiple individual employers. Many PAs find the work rewarding and value the chance to work so directly and responsively with an individual. But there are a number of concerns and difficult issues in managing the employment relationship. UNISON's organising PAs project[1] was set up to deal with a set of common concerns heard from PAs contacting or joining the union:

- isolation – lack of access to support from co-workers or a supervisor;
- pressure to work above and beyond out of a sense of personal obligation and lack of back-up;
- unclear role and relationship boundaries;
- ignorance on the part of both individual employer and worker of mutual employment rights and responsibilities;
- bogus self-employment; that is, attempts to define the arrangement as one of self-employment – stemming sometimes from the worker, sometimes from the individual employer (in some cases, encouraged by information supplied by councils implying that employment versus self-employment is a simple choice) – when the facts do not support this designation;
- lack of resources for training;
- unpaid out-of-pocket expenses such as entry to leisure activities for the PA, as the employer's direct payment does not cover these costs;
- uncertainty about status if the employer is hospitalised, or goes into residential care for short periods;
- difficulties in accessing redundancy rights in the event of an employer's death;
- lack of support for both parties in resolving low-level conflicts.

What comes out of this list of issues is the potential vulnerability and powerlessness of both parties that stems from inadequate support for people entering into this relationship. The potentially precarious nature of the employment relationship has become apparent in the volume of contacts from both parties coming through to ACAS (ACAS, 2013). National newspaper reports of a pensioner allegedly forced to pay £3,500 in redundancy compensation from his own pocket on the death of his wife provide a cautionary tale:

> 'Once the council stopped paying for care direct, people like Dad were made to employ people themselves and then pay them out of the money the council gave them. That means they have a responsibility for PAYE, holiday pay and even redundancy payments. But no-one had made this clear to my father. He had never employed anybody in his life.' (Osborne, 2013)

The UNISON pilot project is focusing on creating networks for PAs and investing union resources to broker access to learning and development and low-level 'managing conflict' training. The project is reaching out to user-led organisations with a strong message around partnership working. However, it is significant that there has been a degree of reservation and concern on the part of some organisations about the prospect of union involvement with PAs. These fears stem from a sense of vulnerability on the part of individual employers and worries that union-organised PAs may make impossible demands. This is in part because the pay and conditions individual employers are able to offer, and the degree to which they able to comply with statutory and good employment practice, is so dependent on the value of the direct payments they receive from the local authority.

In practice, there is no simple shift of power to users. It is a complex situation where the two main parties may end up with responsibility but not much power, while a third party, the local authority, continues to exercise power through its control over the purse strings. These issues require a national settlement and understanding about what level of training and what kind of pay and conditions are needed to ensure good quality care and support. In the early days of personalisation, there was great resistance to any national policy prescription. It is interesting to note that calls to consider measures such as mandatory underpinning of PA rates of pay – measures that UNISON has long called for – are now coming from a diverse range of perspectives as organisations grapple with how to make things work better on the ground (ADASS et al, 2013).

Encouraging a shift in responsibility for employer liabilities from care providers to service users was designed to shift power so that service users could deploy and direct their care worker with full autonomy rather than be restricted by permitted tasks offered by care providers. The question of whether control can be achieved without users taking on all the legal and financial responsibilities of employment, but giving them a more active role within the care agency, has not been fully explored in the UK.

A UNISON study trip to Sweden observed a well-established personal assistance sector where individual direct employment was not much in evidence. People qualifying for state funding for personal assistance had three routes open to them: they could recruit a PA who would then become an employee of the Swedish municipality, but deployed to work with them directly; they could join a cooperative and the PA they recruited would then become an employee of the co-operative and benefit from collectively negotiated pay and conditions; or they could recruit a PA who would be employed via an agency. Very few people opted to become individual employers.

Conclusion

Personal budgets were conceived as the means by which power could be taken from the workforce and given to the user – a zero-sum game. In practice, the narrative of user empowerment through worker disempowerment has proved to be over-simplistic. It is becoming increasingly clear that this power shift has not happened in the way that was envisaged. That is because the dynamics of power involved are complex, reflecting conflicting priorities for the distribution of resources and the marketisation of care provision with power mediated through the processes of commissioning and contracting out.

A combination of spending cuts and failure to develop a nationally coordinated and comprehensive workforce strategy means that greater disempowerment of both users and the workforce is where we may end up. Increasing restrictions on the value of personal budgets are severely curtailing practitioners' scope to engage in creative support planning. Direct payments are falling short of the amount needed to cover decent employment conditions. This means low pay, job insecurity, lack of access to training and poor prospects for care and support workers. And that means high turnover and fractured relationships for users. These are the challenges that need to be addressed if the ideals of personalisation are to be salvaged from the implementation quagmire.

Survey evidence shows continuing support among practitioners for the ideals of user personalisation (Community Care et al, 2010, 2011, 2012, 2013). But we need to reject the divide-and-rule narrative of workers with too much power and concentrate instead on empowerment for both workers and service users. This needs to happen across the spectrum – from practitioners able to sign off budgets and care plans, to homecare workers with greater discretion over the activities they complete and the time they spend with service users. This does not necessarily need to be mediated through the personal budget transaction. But it does need more training and support for workers to work innovatively and collaboratively, a reversal of the marketisation of care provision and more investment to make care and support work a viable and attractive career choice.

Note

[1] This project began in 2013 with the aim of developing support networks for PAs along with learning and development opportunities. The project is testing union-organising models that can accommodate the unique features of PA working. An early achievement has been the establishment of an on-

line resource where PAs can network with each other, get information about training opportunities and access relevant news and advice (www.pa-unison. org.uk).

TWELVE

A view from social work practice

Victoria Hart

What does 'personalisation' mean to me as a social worker who has been working in adult and mental health services for about ten years? It means a lot less to me now than it meant when the new language burst onto the scene in the mid-2000s. When I first started working with direct payments in adult social care, it was liberating and exciting. Contrary to some of the murmurings at the time, we, as social work practitioners, wanted people to be able to have the best quality care, which was tailored towards them. Having a professional qualification infers some skills and knowledge, but it never made or makes me an expert on the preferences of the people I work with. I became used to assessing needs based on forms and formulas, but sometimes the provision of services seemed to be lacking in terms of flexibility, choice and quality. These new policy drives were exciting – they allowed people to choose the providers they wanted and employ personal assistants whom they chose rather than forfeiting themselves to the block contracted care provided by the local authority. It was a win–win situation. There was little impact on the costs to the local authority, but the quality of care and the ethos of choice were improved for those who accessed them.

Yes, there was additional paperwork but the result was generally a highly satisfying piece of work where people we worked with were put at the forefront of choosing their own care, prioritising the needs that they felt should be met, despite what professionals might tell them. It was, and still can be, a liberating way to work that promotes real empowerment rather than the 'empowerment' that is granted by professional gift. It was social work. Maybe not the 'old-fashioned, community-based social work' that was eulogised by our lecturers whose practice was fixed at least ten years behind current policy, but it felt like it was the right thing to do.

The idea that the scope of direct payments would grow through personalisation was an exciting one. After I qualified as a social worker, I worked primarily with older people and this was a group of people who received far less funding than working-age adults with physical and learning disabilities. Older people and people with mental health needs had been excluded to a large extent from participating fully in the first waves of direct payments, so the hope was that the new agenda, when it arose, would take the research evidence that had been gathered when direct payments were being used and focus on those groups where there had been the slowest uptake and where there were more complex issues related to capacity to manage or determine budgets and care and where people did not have informal support networks of family and friends on tap to offer support.

Looking back now, I can see we were always being set up for a fall. The problem was, and still is, that the rhetoric over-promised and has under-delivered, and that leads to disillusionment with the processes and formalities that are behind co-production in principle. How can we call personalisation co-production, when the drivers behind it have excluded so many and seem to continually be asking the same groups of people the same questions without looking beyond at solving some of the identified difficulties such as access, availability and quality of care?

I'm loath to critique what is the inherently great policy aim of involving people in choice and more flexible care, not least because there has been an agenda from policymakers to lay much of the blame for poor implementation on disgruntled practitioners. However, it's hard not to want to shout some of the failings and disillusionment from the rooftops in order for the problems that exist to be identified and to stop the same problems from being overlooked again. We tried to raise these problems at the time, as practitioners, but were constantly rebuffed by disheartening statements claiming it was our fault that the policy was not working. We, as social work practitioners, were an easy target for organisations that were paid to ensure that policies were implemented. It felt and still feels like a betrayal – not for social workers, we can live with that – but for people who rely on these policies to work.

Looking from the bottom up at the people who write and develop policies and guidance, I have spent more than a few hours wondering if they have ever listened to practitioners on the ground, away from their well-defined focus groups, and listened to the issues we have raised regarding the less vocal groups of people that we work with. I hear lots of jargon – personalisation, person-centred support, resource allocation systems, 'Making it Real' – and I think, after 20 years of working in social care, if I struggle to understand them without a glossary, how are we, as a sector managing to make anything at all real, in terms of promoting flexible ways of people having more say over the services they receive?

The language of personalisation needs to be accessible and open. We need to find something other than 'personalisation' to describe it for a start, as the word has become redundant, meaningless, and indeed toxic, in terms of not meaning what it says. Those who are driving the agenda from the government need to drop their impermeable defensiveness and positive vibes to understand what is really happening on the ground – not only with those who actively engage with these agendas and choose to join user-led groups but also – and even more so – with those who don't know how and who to access to be involved. The lack of engagement with professionals and the isolation by means of criticism of social workers, who try to do the best they can with poor tools and within time constraints that are excessive, has been a real failure of those who have been charged with 'leading' personalisation into the light of a universally accessible change in policy.

So where did it go wrong?

I'm not an academic or a manager with strategic oversight. I am someone who has worked with people with advanced dementias for many years, many of whom have had no family local to them or families who are not able to provide support in terms of managing budgets. I have seen groups of people I work with actively excluded from the agenda as I've seen it.

For working-age adults and those who are fully engaged and interested in the process of employing people themselves, where there is a pool of experienced and skilled employees, I have seen enormous positive changes and gains in the quality of life on the basis of having personal budgets and more say in the process of change. The positive stories often come from people who have been very engaged in the process of organising and managing their own care, or within learning disabilities services where the funding is higher, and often families may be more involved in helping put together and managing packages of care for their children.

For older adults, and for people who have cognitive impairments to the extent that they are not able to make decisions about their own care or manage the finances to become employers, I have seen little change. We have moved people to 'personal budgets' rather than directly purchased care, but these have been no different from the directly purchased care that was in place previously. Yes, they tick the box on the local authority performance indicator that says that Mrs Smith is now getting a personal budget, but Mrs Smith has the same carers from the same block-purchased and approved care agency, providing the same tasks on a care plan with the same time allowed. Yet, to the local authority and to the government, that is personalisation 'done'. Yet, Mrs Smith isn't getting the same standard and level of service as Mr Brown, who is actively involved in managing his own direct payment and has employed a personal assistant directly, who meets his needs, and whom he pays less to because he doesn't need to take account of the agency fees that Mrs Smith pays. Who is getting the better service? I think we would agree that Mr Brown is – yet they both tick the 'personalisation' box.

It is this dishonesty that is difficult to manage as a practitioner. We now have a two-tier system where those who are able to manage their own budgets or who have support to do so receive a 'gold standard' service. This is the type of service we would like everyone to receive, but people with the greatest needs or those who don't have family to support them in managing the inherent employment and budgeting tasks, or who lack the capacity to do so, receive a second-rate service delivered in the same way as before. Unless policymakers address these inequalities in the provision of care – something they have known about for many, many years – there will be no genuine 'personalisation' and the policy agenda will be seen as a scam by people who work within the field.

The roll-out of personal budgets for all, whether managed by an individual, their representative or the local authority, is a fantastic ideal to work towards, but working in the field has engendered a cynicism that renders some of the language to be laughable. We have been tasked with additional administration with less time available in which to do it, and been given tools that seem to chase the ideal of person-centred care away. If we look at the processes of assessment and access into the 'adult social care' system, there may be a self-assessment process that will automatically screen out some groups of people who don't feel comfortable laying all the 'weaknesses' out on a form to await assistance. Because of the nature of the conditions of those I worked with – mainly dementias – I provided help with these assessments. The assessment was akin to a benefits form based on highlighting people's deficits and things that need 'fixing'. 'Do you have any problems with your continence?', 'Do you need any help to go to the shops?' – these questions create stigma and distance in themselves. The answers are then used to 'score' points as a part of the resource allocation system. The flaws in these systems in terms of how they gather points to make budgets are covered in detail elsewhere in this book.

It should be understood, though, that it is disheartening as a professional to imagine that this is what is meant by 'personalisation'.

After a budget had been attributed, we would be asked to plan support around people's needs if they were not looking at a direct payment – which was the case with most of the people I worked with. While I'd love to claim I had time to lovingly craft person-centred care plans, in the pace of the job I had, it was rarely something I was able to do. If there were families involved who could help, that was a bonus, but otherwise it was a task that was added on to the rest of day with no protected time to be more creative.

As for being innovative, the difficulties come in the distance between the rhetoric and the reality. While the shiny policy brochures are all about user choice – local leisure centres versus day centres, for example – the reality, in my experience, often came down to a choice between one shower a day or two baths a week, all because of the levels of funding we had to 'play' with. There was little 'allowed' for anything other than the core personal care tasks within older adults' services and while, yes, there could be some leeway in determining which agency to use, it still came down to cost. Our specialist dementia service, for example, cost double the amount of a local private agency that paid its workers minimum wage, so decisions about one hour from a specialist carer versus two from a non-specialist are more likely to be the real decisions made rather than decisions about who is going to provide the best care.

To the future

I try to be hopeful and think that there will be more opportunities for people who have been excluded by the rush towards more choice to be better engaged and involved in the processes that will provide equity of access to quality services. If I were in a more senior position than I am, I would ask those who are engaged in policy design and research to look actively at the areas where we know that the policy is not working and try to speak to people, families and practitioners to identify the challenges and design systems better. I would embed independent advocacy in the resource allocation system processes for people who may lack the capacity to engage in the process of choosing and employing their own care team. I would change the language to make it understandable. I would change processes to make them transparent in terms of understanding and knowing when a cut in budget means a cut in budget and not a pretence of choice. I would try to engage with local people and services to build up capacity among people who are going to be employed to provide care because you can give people budgets, but if no one is available to employ, it won't help.

There is no use just talking to the Association of Directors of Adult Social Services and 'leaders' in the Department of Health about what is going wrong and the fixation on process rather than result. They devise policies – they are not involved with implementing them. I hope that the future will be about engaging and involving social workers rather than isolating and excluding them. This policy needs to work for people who are dependent on good social care but it can't happen when the blame is flung without thought.

The way through the murky water is to promote a culture of trust, honesty and responsiveness among people who use services, their families and carers, and those in local authorities and in the voluntary sector who work on the coal face of health and in social care, visiting clients every day. Nothing would make me happier than a system of choice and control that provides better quality of care for everyone, but we have to acknowledge that there's a long way to go and we all have to listen harder.

Part Four
Personalisation in the NHS: personal health budgets

THIRTEEN

Managing a personal health budget: Malcolm's story(book)

Colin Royle

Since receiving a personal health budget in 2009, my dad's medication has been reduced by two-thirds, he now receives more consistency in his care, he no longer requires the support of a care manager or a consultant, and he now gets to choose where and when his care is provided, and by whom. It isn't so much that receiving a personal health budget has changed our lives; it is more that it has helped to restore them.

In hindsight my dad, Malcolm, first began suffering with dementia in 2005. All of his life he had been an outgoing, hard-working and thoughtful individual. Yet suddenly, elements of his personality started disappearing.

It was leading up to his retirement that he first started displaying what, on reflection, were the first symptoms of right frontal lobe dementia. Malcolm had always been a very confident individual, doing various public speaking gigs and socialising at every opportunity. He had always taken life in his stride, yet in the November of 2005 he started suffering with panic attacks.

Unusual as it was, nothing much was thought of it at first. His life was about to undergo a massive transformation brought about by his retirement. He had worked full-time since the age of 16 and now, at 60 years of age, he was ultimately taking a step into the unknown. It was only natural that he should feel slightly uneasy about it.

Standing at six feet tall, 13 stone in weight and at only 60 years of age, Malcolm didn't represent what one may consider to be your typically old and frail dementia patient. Yet in the January of 2006, his weight suddenly dropped to just 11 stone in a matter of weeks.

Despite his weight gradually returning, we noticed a huge loss in confidence and change in his demeanour. The outgoing, approachable demeanour he had always displayed had gone and he now appeared somewhat insular. Suddenly, he looked terrified of talking to people.

Such symptoms continued over the following months, yet it was difficult to identify something tangible to take to the doctors to evidence our concerns. But by the summer of 2006, we were at least acknowledging the changes as a family.

As the symptoms persisted, we gradually encouraged my dad to seek support, and by the summer of 2007, he had seen two different doctors, a mental health worker, a social worker and a memory clinician, none of whom spotted any signs or symptoms that pointed to anything other than a difficulty in adjusting to retirement.

It was difficult for the professionals involved; after all, they only got a sound-bite into who Malcolm really is. But we as a family knew my dad, and we *knew* something wasn't right. The first doctor we had seen had initially suspected dementia after listening to our concerns. We had hoped with all our hearts that it wasn't dementia, yet each time we were seen and ultimately turned away by one of numerous professionals, we left feeling more concerned than relieved.

Unfortunately, by the February of 2008, his symptoms and behaviours had increased to such a level that he had to be placed under section 3 of the Mental Health Act 2007. He was to remain in hospital for the next six months.

The ward on which my dad was 'housed' consisted of various people with numerous mental health concerns, ranging from schizophrenia and bipolar disorder to younger people with early onset dementia such as my dad. While it was a relief that a more in-depth analysis into Malcolm's behaviour would now take place, his reaction to this environment was concerning.

My dad began emulating the various behaviours of other patients on the ward, and, ultimately, his own needs increased at an alarming rate. By the summer of 2008, his behaviours were becoming increasingly aggressive, and less and less predictable.

A diagnosis had eventually been determined and we were told that he suffered from right frontal lobe dementia, a very rare form of the disease. This explained why his behaviours were less typical than with other forms of dementia, such as Alzheimer's. We spoke to Professor Neary at Manchester Hope Hospital, who had pioneered much of the research into this disease, and we discussed what the future may hold.

There had been a presumption by the professionals involved in my dad's care that he would move into a care home after being discharged from hospital. Due to the unpredictability of his behaviours and the dangers he now presented to both himself and others, he met the Continuing Healthcare criteria, so any package of care that he was to receive would be funded by the NHS. However, after seeing such deterioration in Malcolm's condition during his stay in hospital, in

August 2008, we decided as a family that we wished for my dad to spend his life at home.

Many within the care industry were sceptical of my abilities to look after my father, a man with so many complex needs. After all, I had no formal training as a doctor, or a nurse or a psychiatrist. Still, we pointed out that, as a family, we had been the most consistent factors in my dad's care to date. We had identified the changes in my dad's behaviours over the two years before he received a diagnosis. And the staff at the hospital themselves acknowledged how much more amenable my dad was to the requests of his family than he was to those of the hospital staff. Despite our lack of 'qualifications', we too wanted to be acknowledged as experts in my dad's care. So a decision was made.

I took on the responsibility of becoming my dad's full-time carer. It was apparent at this time that there was a serious short-fall in support available from the NHS. We were presented with just one option – for my dad to attend a day centre for four days a week, Monday to Thursday, 8am to 5pm. It was then that I first enquired about the possibility of having a direct payment, something that I knew existed in social care. Unfortunately, we were told that this was not possible, as it was illegal to receive money provided by the NHS in such a way.

Due to the intense nature of caring for my father, I had to give up my career and instead work a part-time job during the hours that my dad attended the day centre. However, after around nine months of looking after my dad and his increasing needs on a full-time basis, we recognised that the current package of care was unsustainable.

The day centre was not fulfilling my dad's needs. Due to low rates of pay, there was a high turnover of staff, and therefore a lack of consistency in my dad's care. Much of the training that the staff received was Alzheimer's specific, but with my dad's condition being a rare form of dementia, he presented very differently from anything they had been trained to deal with. The activities at the day centre were also very generic, and none of them interested my dad.

Nine months since first attending the day centre, my dad's medication had been tripled, his anxieties were continuing to increase and the professional involvement in my dad's package was escalating. He also frequently verbalised how he wished to stop attending the day centre and spend more time at home.

As a family we were also struggling. There was no flexibility in the hours during which the care package could be received. I had not had an evening off since my dad came home in the August, and was exhausted. Something needed to change.

Thankfully we were approached by our social worker about the prospect of having a personal health budget (PHB). It was explained that the idea behind a PHB was to allow more choice and control over the care that we received. The budget was to be set at a rate equivalent to the cost of my dad going into a care home, as had been anticipated some months earlier.

The process of actually getting a personal health budget was a difficult one. Blackburn, where we lived, was not one of the Department of Health pilot sites, so we couldn't receive our budget as a direct payment. Thankfully, we were put in contact with Jo Fitzgerald, who was one of the first people in the country to go through the process, as she managed a personal health budget for her son, Mitchell.

Such peer support felt extremely useful to us as a family, as it gave us an opportunity to explore ways in which we could use our budget with somebody who had their own experience of having one, and who also offered her expertise without an agenda. Like us, Jo also recognised people as experts in their own lives, and saw personal health budgets as a way of tapping into such knowledge. With Jo's support, we linked up with a third party – Crossroads Ribble Valley – a charity and care provider that offered to hold the budget on our behalf. We discussed what support we felt might be useful from them and how this might be provided. It was important to us as a family to retain as much choice and control as possible.

Unfortunately, my dad was no longer capable of actively making decisions, so I took on the responsibility of advocating on his behalf. We agreed with Crossroads that any decisions around who to employ, rates of pay and what hours people worked would be made by the family. Crossroads would provide advice around employment law, managing the money and any support requested with regard to staff recruitment or disciplinary matters.

When recruiting, we felt that it was important to set our own rates of pay so that we could retain staff and ultimately provide more consistency in my dad's package of care. A rate was set that was substantially higher than the national minimum wage received by the staff at the day centre. Although this ultimately reduced the number of hours in my dad's care package, we made the decision that quality of care was more important than quantity.

Over the months leading into 2010, we recruited four members of staff while gradually reducing the hours my dad spent at the day centre. Allowing Malcolm to spend more time at home was something that was important to all of us, particularly him. By receiving his care in this manner, his entire care package could be tailored around his own needs, and not designed to fit in with the needs of other service users.

My dad now had the option of sleeping in between Monday and Thursday, and could also use support in the evening if there was an activity he wished to do. He had choice over who provided his care and the members of staff that we employed. He could spend his time doing things that he chose to do, such as going for walks, or feeding the ducks, or going to the cinema. It was 'person-centred planning' at its best.

What we also noticed as a family was the change in relationship between ourselves and the professionals involved in my dad's care. No longer were we attending appointments and our opinions being overlooked. Instead, we were now being treated as the experts we were with regard to my dad's condition and his ever-changing behaviours. We were also being given a lot of flexibility and opportunity to be creative in the way that we used my dad's budget.

We used his PHB to purchase a digital TV package. My dad was finding adverts increasingly difficult to cope with due to the loud noises used to get viewers' attention. The digital TV package enabled us to record his favourite TV shows such as quiz programmes, football and his favourite films. He could now watch them when he liked and without adverts, reducing his anxieties, and in turn his unpredictable behaviours, and ultimately keeping him safe.

My dad was thriving under his new package of care. Within 18 months of receiving a personal health budget, his medication had been reduced by two-thirds and any need for input from care managers or consultants had dissipated. Unfortunately, dementia is a degenerative disease and my dad's condition will continue to get worse. What a personal health budget has allowed him to do, however, is get the most out of the life that he has left and live it in the dignified way that he deserves.

FOURTEEN

Evaluation of the personal health budget pilot programme[1]

Julien Forder and Karen Jones

Personalisation and consumer direction are well-established policy initiatives in long-term care (OECD, 2005). With close links to long-term (social) care, these measures are also being considered for health-related support for people with long-term conditions. In 2009, the Department of Health (DH) in England announced a pilot programme to explore the use of personal health budgets (PHBs) for people with long-term health conditions such as chronic obstructive pulmonary disease (COPD), diabetes, mental health, and also for people likely to have significant co-morbidities using NHS Continuing Healthcare services. The underlying rationale was similar to that expounded in long-term care initiatives. Personalisation was viewed as a mechanism to encourage choice and control among individuals who use services, which in turn would have the possibility to control increasing costs.

The potential scope of these initiatives in healthcare is substantial. The DH in England estimated that around 15 million people in England (30% of the population) have at least one long-term health condition, accounting for 70% of the health and social care budget (DH, 2012d). In addition to the costs that can be attributed to long-term health conditions, there is a significant impact on people's lives that also needs to be considered (DH, 2012d). The personalisation agenda acknowledges this impact by putting individuals at the centre of all decisions made about them, with the aim of giving them greater choice and control over how services are managed. It has been suggested by the DH that personalisation, information, choice, supported self-care, shared decision making and service integration will become the norm for people with a long-term health condition (DH, 2012d).

In the healthcare system, personal health budgets are viewed as one mechanism to achieve the aim of giving people greater choice and control by offering a new way of managing services to meet health needs. Three distinct principles underlie personal health budgets: following assessment a budget is made known to the patient before the support/care planning stage; patients are encouraged to play a central role in the support/care planning process; and patients can choose how they would like to manage their personal health budget (DH, 2009c).

To explore the impact that personal health budgets can have on health and social care outcomes, the DH commissioned a three-year evaluation that ran alongside the pilot programme of the initiative (DH, 2009c). The overall aim of the evaluation was to identify whether personal health budgets deliver better health and care outcomes when compared with conventional service delivery; and, if so, to identify the most effective implementation process. Of the 64 pilot sites involved in piloting personal health budgets, 20 sites were selected to be in-depth evaluation sites, with the remainder being wider-cohort sites. The in-depth sites recruited individuals with one of the following health conditions: long-term conditions (including COPD, diabetes and long-term neurological conditions); mental health; stroke; and individuals receiving NHS Continuing Healthcare (Forder et al, 2012).

A further aim of the evaluation was to explore whether the way personal health budgets were introduced in the pilot sites had an impact on outcomes and costs. A range of different implementations of personal health budgets were used in the pilots with differences in how budgets were assessed and determined, how they could be used to secure services and support and so on. In all cases, however, mainstream GP and acute services were not covered and continued to be provided outside the personal health budget.

Table 14.1 shows the different ways that personal health budgets were introduced in the sites, varying according to: whether the budget was known before support planning; what flexibility there was in terms of what help could be purchased; and the choice of deployment (including direct payment [DP]). Nineteen of the 20 in-depth pilot sites were classified within one of five implementation models.

During the evaluation (Forder et al, 2012), it was hypothesised that personal health budgets could influence costs and outcomes in four ways:

• they can affect quality of life by improving people's sense of choice and control over their own lives;
• they allow people to change their use of services and support to better match their own needs and preferences, and thereby (indirectly) improving their quality of life;
• they can be set at a higher or lower level than the cost of conventional services they replace;

- they can lead to direct changes in the services actually used; for example, people might use their budget to buy services that might change their demand/need for hospital care.

Table 14.1: Implementation models

Implementation models	In-depth pilot sites
Model 1 Personalised budget is known before support planning Flexibility in what help can be purchased Deployment choice (including DP)	8 pilot sites
Model 2 Budget is known before support planning (but may not be personalised – a set amount) Service directory Deployment choice (including DP)	4 pilot sites
Model 3 Budget is known before support planning (but may not be personalised – a set amount) Lack of flexibility in the help that can be purchased No deployment choice	3 pilot sites
Model 4 Budget is not known before support planning Flexibility in what help can be purchased Variation in the degree of deployment choice	4 pilot sites
Model 5 Model 1 and 2 combined	12 pilot sites

The evaluation (Forder et al, 2012) compared the experience of just over 1,000 people selected to receive personal health budgets (PHB group) with around 1,000 continuing with conventional support arrangements (control group). To investigate the impact of personal health budgets on outcomes, participants were invited to participate in a face-to-face interview within one month of gaining informed consent and again 12 months later. The interviews explored a number of outcome measures including the following:

- Health-related quality of life: the EQ-5D utility scale aims to measure a person's quality of life in domains likely to be related to their underlying health status. It measures personal functioning (as potentially constrained by poor health). The three-level version was used.

- Care-related quality of life: the Adult Social Care Outcomes Toolkit (ASCOT) was used to explore the achievement of activities of daily living that might come from the support of services and interventions, as well as from personal functioning (Netten et al, 2012).
- Psychological wellbeing: the 12-item version of the General Health Questionnaire (Goldberg, 1992) was used. It explores whether respondents have experienced a particular symptom or behaviour over the past few weeks.

The interviews also collected information about community and primary care service use. In addition, demographic and socioeconomic information was collected, as well as information about current circumstances.

Participants' health condition, clinical indicators (HbA1C for patients with diabetes or lung-function [forced expiratory volume] test for patients with COPD) and their use of primary healthcare services were gathered from GP records. Secondary care service use data was extracted from the Hospital Episodes Statistics (Health and Social Care Information Centre). Both sets of data were collected at two time-points during the study period: first, around the time of consent in order to compare the previous 12 months' activity; second, around 12 months after recruitment to gather information for the year following consent.

The study was designed to accommodate a difference-in-difference method whereby the relevant experiences of people in the personal health budget group could be compared with those in the control group, after accounting for any difference in their situation before the intervention (the PHB) was used. To this end, relevant data was collected about study participants at baseline (that is, before the PHB process began and after the consent date) and at follow-up (around 12 months after consent). This method aims to ensure that any remaining differences between the groups at follow-up are due to the use of PHBs. Multiple regression was also used with a range of control factors to account for any differences between groups at baseline that might affect any change over time in their outcomes and costs beyond any true effect of personal health budgets.

The impact of personal health budgets on quality of life

The use of personal health budgets was associated with a significant improvement in both care-related quality of life and psychological wellbeing of patients over the 12-month follow-up period relative to those receiving conventional services. Supporting the view that personal health budgets should focus on improving the daily management of a condition rather than affect health status per se, the evaluation did not find a significant impact on health-related quality of life (EQ-5D). This indicator aims to measure wellbeing in domains that are related to underlying health conditions, which would not be expected to change over the follow-up period for people using PHBs. Furthermore, the evaluation did not show that personal health budgets had an impact on the clinical indicator for patients with either diabetes (HbA1C) or COPD (lung-function test). The findings suggest that the benefits of personal health budgets stemmed from the value that people placed on having increased choice and control in their lives, and the capacity this gave them to improve the more complex or higher-order aspects of their quality of life (Forder et al, 2012).

The impact of personal health budgets on costs and cost-effectiveness

A principal aim of the evaluation of the personal health budget pilot programme (Forder et al, 2012) was to explore whether the initiative could have an impact on outcomes at an acceptable cost. At the time of the pilot programme, this was high on the political agenda in the context of fiscal austerity. Following the pilot programme and evaluation, the focus turned more towards sustainability – as Clinical Commissioning Groups would need to work within current financial constraints (Audit Commission, 2012b). In terms of costs, the evaluation found that for both the personal health budget and control groups there was a pattern of increasing direct costs and falling indirect costs over the follow-up period. Expenditure to meet direct costs (that is, the costs of social care, wellbeing, nursing and therapy, and other health services) increased by 25% over the period for the control group and 20% for the personal health budget group, on average. Indirect costs (GP services, hospital care), however, fell by 33% for the personal health budget group compared with 18% for the control group, on average. In both cases, the main reduction was for hospital services rather than primary care (GP services). A reduction in secondary care costs often results from a 'regression to the mean', in other words when recruitment to a programme involves participants using a lot of secondary care services that subsequently reduce to more normal levels during the study period. By including a control group and using a difference-in-difference method, this spurious effect should have been avoided in this study.

With regard to the total costs of services and support used by all study participants (that is, direct and indirect costs), the analysis found that total costs increased, on average, by £1,920 per person over the study period in the control group and by £800 in the personal health budget group (a net reduction of £1,120 for the personal health budget group compared with the control group on average). However, due to the high level of variation of costs between study participants, these net cost differences between the personal health budget and control groups were not statistically significant.

Personal health budgets would be cost-effective relative to conventional service delivery if they produced greater net monetary benefits (NMB) than this usual care comparator. Benefits are the £-value of improvements in care-related quality of life. Following the approach used in England by the National Institute for Health and Care Excellence (NICE), an implicit value of between £20,000 and £30,000 is assessed for an improvement of one quality-adjusted year of life (QALY) (NICE, 2007; Raftery, 2009). Net monetary benefit was calculated as the value of any improvement in quality of life associated with PHBs relative to those in the control group less the difference in cost between the two groups. A difference between the groups (after controlling for baseline differences) in NMB of greater than zero signifies cost-effectiveness. It is an alternative way to express that PHBs have additional costs of less than a cost-effectiveness threshold of between £20,000 and £30,000 additional cost per QALY gained. Currently, there is no established cost-effectiveness valuation for the ASCOT measure, although, given the equivalent anchoring to death as for EQ-5D, a similar value was inferred, that is, £30,000 in the main case.

Using care-related quality of life (ASCOT), personal health budgets showed greater benefit and less cost, on average, than conventional services. In particular, personal health budgets were cost-effective (in having a greater NMB than the control group, after baseline control) at the 10% significance level. Sensitivity analysis supported this result, suggesting if anything that PHBs are cost-effective at 5% significance levels. In the case of using health-related quality of life (EQ-5D), personal health budgets showed greater net benefits compared with conventional services, but these were not statistically significant.

A number of analyses were performed on sub-groups of the main study population (for example, by people with different health conditions). Sub-group effects were estimated using the difference between NMB gain for the people with personal health budgets in the sub-group and the people recruited to the control group in the same sub-group (ensuring like-with-like comparisons of experience of personal health budgets or the usual care process for these sub-populations). A particular focus was on the impact of personal health budgets for those people in the NHS Continuing Healthcare cohort. Using the ASCOT scale, the results indicated that personal health budgets were cost-effective for both NHS Continuing Healthcare and mental health cohorts at the 10% significance level (Forder et al, 2012).

Implementation and the impact on outcomes/cost-effectiveness

The evaluation found (through sub-group analysis) that the implementation process had a significant bearing on cost-effectiveness. When the PHB was implemented following the main principles as outlined by the DH (2009c) and classified as following Model 1 (see Table 14.1, as previously reported), personal health budgets were shown to be cost-effective when considering care-related quality of life (ASCOT) relative to conventional service delivery. However, when personal health budgets were implemented in the way that was least consistent with policy intentions (Model 3), it was found that personal health budgets were not cost-effective compared with conventional service delivery (Forder et al, 2012).

Conclusion

In conclusion, a range of measures of outcome or effectiveness was included within the evaluation to build up a comprehensive picture of the potential impact of personal health budgets. However, there were a number of limitations to this highly complex evaluation as outlined in the final report that should be acknowledged when interpreting the finding (Forder et al, 2012). In particular, conducting a full randomised controlled trial was not feasible, and therefore there was not a way to make the evaluation 'blind' in the sense that participants would not know whether they were in the personal health budget or control groups. Furthermore, the evaluation had to deal with the design tension between allowing sufficient elapsed time after baseline for the effects of personal health budgets to be felt on the one hand and minimising loss to follow-up on the other. There was a degree of missing data in the analysis, which was addressed using multiple-imputation methods. Nonetheless, these methods involve certain assumptions which could affect the results. As a consequence, the study used a wide range of predictors in the statistical imputation models to estimate values for missing data, and also used different specifications of the imputation model to assess the sensitivity of the results to the implicit assumptions of those models.

Despite these limitations, the evaluation was able to provide support for the national roll-out of personal health budgets that was announced during the pilot programme. On 4 October 2011, the Secretary of State for Health announced that, subject to the evaluation, by April 2014 everyone in receipt of NHS Continuing Healthcare would have the right to ask for a personal health budget (DH, 2012e). A further announcement followed that highlighted that people receiving NHS Continuing Healthcare would have the right to have a personal health budget as from October 2014.

Note

[1] The evaluation of the personal health budget pilot programme was commissioned and funded by the Policy and Strategy Directorate in the DH. The views expressed are not necessarily those of the DH.

The evaluation team combined the expertise of researchers at the Personal Social Services Research Unit at the University of Kent, the Social Policy Research Unit at the University of York, the Department of Social Policy at the London School of Economics and Political Science and at Imperial College London.

FIFTEEN

Personal health budgets: a threat to the NHS?

Colin Slasberg

When Norman Lamb, Minister for Care and Support, announced to Parliament the introduction of a right to ask for a personal health budget (Lamb, 2013), he said it would "... go further towards our goal of providing greater personalisation within our NHS".

He thus saw a personal health budget (PHB) as a means to an end, not an end in itself. By not declaring any alternative definition of the word 'personalisation', we can deduce that he was applying the word in its common usage. The *Oxford English Dictionary* defines the word as 'designing something to meet someone's requirements'.

The NHS reminds us that the founding principles of the NHS were and remain (NHS Choices, 2013):

- that it meet the needs of everyone;
- that it be free at the point of delivery;
- that it be based on clinical need, not ability to pay.

Personalisation, understood in the common sense of the word, poses no threat to these principles. On the contrary, there is an argument that the 'one-size-fits-all' delivery systems into which people have to fit – the antithesis of personalisation – contravene the principles, as the service provided to the person is not based on their real needs.

There is, however, a serious question as to whether the Minister is right in claiming that PHBs will promote personalisation. His confidence has two sources. The first is social care, which has been delivering personal budgets (PBs) since 2008. Sector and political leaders believe that PBs are such a certain route to personalisation that the terms are used interchangeably. The president of the Association of Directors of Adult Social Services (ADASS, 2013b), responding to the news that the target for the number of people said to have a personal budget by 2013 (70%) had been met said that the service was now 'providing personalised social care services to well over two thirds of eligible individuals'.

The second source of information for the Minister is the evaluation of the PHB pilots, where people said to have a PHB enjoyed better outcomes than a control group that did not.

However, this chapter will set out the evidence that wrong lessons are being drawn and that the Minister's confidence is misplaced. If the NHS stays on its current course, PHBs will both fail to deliver personalisation and will undermine its founding principles. The chapter will also outline how PHBs might be re-envisioned to deliver personalisation for all.

What is a personal health budget?

NHS guidance (NHS England, 2013) sets out the PHB process as:

- making contact;
- understanding the person's health and wellbeing needs;
- working out the amount of money available;
- making a care plan;
- organising care and support;
- monitoring and review.

This replicates the key elements of the PB process in social care. The innovative element is the allocation of money before care planning. This is to achieve a shift in control from professional to the person, so enabling the person choice over the content of the care plan. The Association of Directors of Adult Social Services describes a personal budget as 'a clear, upfront amount of funding from adult social care which individuals can spend on the services and support they need' (ADASS, 2013b). In social care this process is called self-directed support.

The national evaluation of the PHB pilots: drawing the wrong lessons

The evaluation of the three-year pilots (Forder et al, 2012) has been taken as evidence that this approach to PHBs worked. There was clear evidence that people in the PHB group enjoyed better outcomes than the control group. In its response to the evaluation (DH, 2012f), the government said that it showed PHBs to be '... cost effective when implemented as the policy intended and patients have genuine control.'

This view reflects the responses of proponents of self-directed support. Julie Stansfield, Chief Executive of In Control, the organisation credited with creating self-directed support, in an article for *The Guardian* (Stansfield, 2013), said of the evaluation: 'Crucially, the findings about what works replicated those in social care. To achieve the best results, personal budgets must be delivered according to the principles of self-directed support'.

However, this is not what the evaluation actually found. The pilot sites were divided into four groups. One group (consisting of 225 people, 19.2% of all those with a PHB) were not offered an up-front allocation. However, this group still enjoyed the best outcomes of those with a PHB. Conversely, one of the three other groups that did claim to offer an up-front allocation (206 people, comprising 17.6% of the sample) did not achieve better outcomes. The evaluation team came to the following conclusion (Forder et al, 2012, p 76): '... possibly that it is the greater choice and flexibility that is more important than knowing the budget level'.

Social care: drawing the wrong lessons

There is mounting evidence that the impact of PBs is not as ADASS believes. At the heart of the problem is the way the up-front allocation works. Allocating money before knowing the cost of meeting needs raises both legal and financial risks. For this reason, it was made 'indicative' only, with the amount of resource to be decided following care planning. This led Series and Clements (2013) to question what function it actually has. Slasberg and colleagues (2013) report that Freedom of Information requests to more than 50 councils have shown that when councils monitor the difference between the indicative and actual allocations, the ratio of the difference between them is very large. This resonates with the Series and Clements finding, pointing to the actual resource allocation process working quite independently from the indicative budget-setting process.

This raises the rather shocking possibility that, contrary to all public pronouncements, personal budgets, which are defined as an 'up-front' allocation, do not actually exist. Councils are routinely creating an 'indicative budget' as the performance regime requires them to do, but it is playing no part in determining how much people get.

Learning the right lessons from social care

Slasberg and colleagues (2012a) demonstrate that a correct reading of the evidence is that when personalisation and better outcomes do occur, it is only when people take cash as a direct payment. However, this has been the case since direct payments were introduced in 1997. It has allowed people both to create and then manage their own support system, in the main through employment of personal assistants as an alternative to mainstream services. There is no evidence that the central innovation of self-directed support, the up-front allocation, has made any material contribution to their success. The belief that personal budgets are making a difference has been promoted by showcasing the success of those with a direct payment and then claiming them for the personal budget strategy:

- Two national surveys of the strategy (Hatton and Waters, 2011, 2013) assessed the progress of large samples of people said to have a personal budget. However, while in 2011 the percentage of all service users with a direct payment was less than 10%, they comprised 90% of the survey sample. In 2013, while the percentage of all service users with a direct payment had risen to 11%, they comprised 89% of the survey sample.
- There is heavy reliance on personal testimony. While it is only a small minority who take up the direct payment option, there is a sufficiently large pool from which to identify willing contributors.

Are direct payments the answer?

Since 2010, government has made it policy, perhaps in tacit recognition that the PB element was not working, that direct payments should be the default option for service users. This was based on the view that, despite only small numbers taking them up in the 12 years since they were introduced, most if not all could achieve the same benefits by taking a direct payment. This view is encouraged by a body of research that has focused on practitioner and council behaviour required to enable take-up on the premise that their behaviours were the barriers (CSCI, 2004; Hasler, 2013).

The percentage of service users with a direct payment, while still a small minority, has thus more than doubled in the past five years. However, there is reason to believe this target-driven strategy has formed a different cohort of people with a direct payment with no reason to believe they will be achieving better outcomes. Helga Pile (2013, p 56) of UNISON notes that:

> Practitioners responding to a UNISON survey felt that they were implementing a 'one-size-fits-all' approach to personalisation, driven by sign-up targets. This has been exacerbated by the 2010 announcement by government ministers in England that 'direct payments should be the preferred option' for receiving a personal budget. Respondents do not feel that this is real personalisation because the focus is on process not outcomes.

While the original cohort used the cash to purchase and manage their own support system as an alternative to mainstream services, the recent increase in numbers of people with a direct payment has not been associated with a decrease in use of mainstream services. In 2009/10, the amount of home care hours purchased amounted to 183 million, while in 2012/13 it was 187 million (NASCIS, Expenditure and Unit Costs[1]). This resonates with findings that older people who have a direct payment are more likely to use it to purchase mainstream services (Carr, 2013). This suggests that the new cohort is simply taking on the responsibility from the council to carry out the financial transactions with their provider. There is no evidence to believe that using direct payments in this way improves outcomes or personalises the service. Indeed, social care has a long history of people who use their own money to fund social care receiving the same quality of service as those publicly funded (and often paying more for it).

This evidence points to direct payments delivering personalisation only under specific and limited conditions and is not the panacea government hoped it might be.

Flexibility or 'choice and control'?

The PHB guidance (NHS England, 2013) says that the aim of the strategy is to promote 'choice, flexibility and control'. This mixes concepts. Flexibility is the ability to match resource to need. Choice is about control resting with the person so they can make the key decisions. They are different concepts with different policy and practice implications.

A similar confusion has pervaded and damaged social care. Jeff Jerome, then personalisation lead for the Department of Health, speaking to *Community Care* magazine in 2011 in response to concerns that councils were continuing to determine what supports people were getting, said: "I have consistently stressed that there is no requirement for local authorities to restrict how personal budgets ... should be spent. The only conditions are that budgets must be used on things ... that contribute to the meeting of agreed outcomes...." (Dunning, 2011).

If the council believes that the person's choice is either a service that will not meet outcomes the council has agreed, or is one that will meet outcomes the council has not agreed, the council will indeed restrict the service user's choice. It is a statement that professes to support choice, but in reality supports flexibility.

The confusion has arguably resulted in social care taking a backward step in its search for personalisation. Self-directed support is a choice-based model, and its creation has led to a very large, expensive but irrelevant bureaucracy to deliver the redundant up-front allocation (Slasberg et al, 2013). The felony is compounded by a concomitant neglect of the very different challenges to ensure that councils are able to operate flexibly, leaving the majority to continue to receive inflexible services.

The importance of resource levels

In addition to the flexibility that direct payments make possible for those who wish to manage their own support system, there is prima facie evidence that resource levels are also important in achieving better outcomes.

- After ten years of being available, in 2007/08 4.4% of service users with community support had a direct payment (NASCIS, p 2f) yet the percentage of gross spend on direct payments was 7.9% (NASCIS, EX1). The spend per head was thus significantly greater for people with a direct payment.
- Woolham and Benton (2012) compared costs and benefits of a sample of people with a direct payment in a large shire county in 2008/09 with a comparator group. The average value of support packages was 44% greater for people with a direct payment than for the control group.

There is no reason to suppose that the differential is linked to complexity of need, as people with all levels of complexity take a direct payment.

There was prima facie evidence that a similar situation may have existed with the PHB pilots. The mean value of the care packages for PHB holders was £15,100 and for the control group just £11,000. The evaluation team noted that people with more costly packages – the 40% with over £1,000 – were more likely to experience better outcomes. They speculated that the resulting greater flexibility may have been a factor. However, they did not explore whether the differential between the PHB and control groups may have been a factor in the success of the PHB group through them having greater resource relative to need than the control group. They chose to 'infer that the people in the control group are healthier and have lower care needs than the PHB group' (Forder et al, 2012, p 88). While there was indeed some evidence that the differential may have been due in part to different levels of need, there were also indications that there were differential resource levels relative to need.

The Audit Commission (2012b, p 16) found that carrying out assessments in the new way meant that 'pilot sites have found that unmet needs will be identified in care/support planning'. These are needs that would have been met by the pilots that would not be revealed through the conventional processes that the control group experienced.

The evaluation included in-depth interviews with some PHB holders and found that 'the majority appeared satisfied because the amount had allowed them access to the services or items they had felt they needed' (Forder et al, 2012, p 76). The level of satisfaction with resource levels of the control group may not have been similar.

Gadsby (2013, p 21), commenting on the evaluation, says:

> It seems that in many cases, additional resources [in the PHB group] were provided that enabled individuals to pay for extra services or one-off goods. It is perhaps unsurprising, therefore, that overall improvements were found in wellbeing amongst budget holders.

The PHB guidance (NHS England, 2013) states that: 'It is good practice for the budget to cover the full range of health needs' and that the resulting budget 'should always be sufficient to meet the outcomes agreed in the care plan'. It is improbable that current resource levels will permit such a generous level of resourcing in roll-out. Further, such an approach is incompatible with working within a cash-limited budget. The cost of meeting needs is not knowable in advance given that individual needs and the cost of meeting them are unique. Gadsby (2013) reports that a PHB scheme in the Netherlands collapsed due to its failure to control spending.

Implications of these findings for PHBs

If PHBs are to deliver personalisation, they need to be designed to deliver flexibility. This will require the following challenges to be addressed.

- *Free up the resource base.* Flexibility is not possible if the available resource has been spent at the beginning of the year on a limited range of services that work inflexibly. Clinical commissioning groups will need to do two things. First, they must free up enough of their resource base as cash to enable those for whom it is appropriate to go outside of commissioned services to do so. Second, where services are strategically commissioned in advance, this must be done in a way that enables those services to respond flexibly to individual need.
- *Create a framework to enable decisions about fair and appropriate resource allocation within budget.* Assessment of need prior to resource allocation will result in a greater range of needs being identified. A framework will be needed to address the likelihood that even the most cost-effective ways of meeting all needs will exceed the budget. This is both a cultural and technical challenge, but one that cannot be avoided if the Netherlands experience is to be prevented.
- *Develop the skills required for partnership working.* A care plan that is fit for the purpose of meeting an individual's needs in the most cost-effective way requires an accurate understanding of the person's needs and creative thinking about how best to meet them. This calls for the person and practitioner in question to work in partnership, as each has inalienable contributions to make if the care plan is to be fit for purpose.
- *Acknowledge resource levels.* The NHS needs to be clear that the above measures may deliver personalisation within available resources, but that this will not in itself bring about the best levels of health and wellbeing for people. That will also require a sufficient level of resource. A needs-led assessment process will create the information at an individual level to make known the gap between needs and resources. Aggregation will create an information source for strategic planning purposes.

Conclusion

If the government persists with its current course, PHBs will indeed pose a very real threat to the NHS. Some people may well experience better outcomes, but they will be few in number. Better levels of resourcing are likely be a factor in their success, which, within a cash-limited environment, means this will be at the expense of the majority. It will therefore fly in the face of a universal NHS committed to fairness.

If, on the other hand, government re-envisions PHBs as a means to ensure that the right services are matched to the right needs for all, far from posing a threat to the NHS founding principles, it will strengthen and make them relevant to the modern era. The challenges would be significant. It will be a test of the sincerity and resolve of political leaders to move away from the more simple agenda promised them by the choice-based model imported from social care.

Note

[1] All NASCIS (National Adult Social Care Intelligence System) data in this chapter is sourced from https://nascis.hscic.gov.uk/

SIXTEEN

Where next for personal health budgets?

Vidhya Alakeson

Judged by government announcements, the progress of personal health budgets (PHBs) continues apace. Following the government's 2012 announcement that adults and children eligible for NHS Continuing Healthcare (CHC) would be entitled to ask for a PHB from April 2014, a new announcement in 2013 has already transformed the 'right to ask' into a 'right to have' (House of Commons, 2013). However, looking beyond the 56,000 people who are eligible for CHC to the millions with long-term conditions, the future of PHBs looks less certain and straightforward.

The current policy commitment around the roll-out of PHBs beyond CHC is relatively weak; as of 2015, clinical commissioning groups (CCGs) – local purchasers of NHS services – should be able to offer a PHB to anyone with a long-term condition who could benefit (DH, 2012a). For PHBs to become a real option for the many thousands of people with long-term conditions, the NHS will have to confront challenges on three fronts: current approaches to commissioning and reconfiguring services; the lack of clinical awareness and support for PHBs; and the lack of bottom-up demand for PHBs from individuals and families. None of these has presented as significant a challenge in the context of CHC.

Progress will also depend on maintaining the cross-party consensus going forward that has been critical to the development of personalisation to date, as Needham and Glasby discuss in Chapter Two. Here, cracks are emerging that could stall momentum behind PHBs after the next election and even send it into reverse. The value of overcoming these different challenges lies in the demonstrable improvement that PHBs have been shown to make to the wellbeing and quality of life of budget holders in a way that is cost-effective for the NHS (Forder et al, 2012).

PHBs and the challenge for commissioning

A critical question for the future of PHBs is how to fund them on a cost-neutral basis. Estimates suggest that the NHS in England faces a funding gap of £14 billion between 2014/15 and 2021/22, even if funding for the NHS rises in line with GDP growth (Roberts et al, 2012). Issues of financial sustainability were not addressed by the three-year national pilot programme. Many pilot sites funded PHBs by absorbing the costs of providing participants with a PHB at the same time as funding the services they would otherwise have used. These double running costs were feasible for a small number and arguably sensible given the pilot nature of PHBs. Funding PHBs from within existing resources does not present a significant challenge for CHC because care packages are generally already commissioned on an individual basis.

In contrast, funding PHBs for other conditions on a sustainable basis involves two specific commissioning challenges. The first is that many community-based NHS services continue to be commissioned on a block basis with funding tied into existing contracts. Releasing this funding to provide PHBs on a cost-neutral basis is difficult because there are no clear prices for the different services provided within the contract, let alone prices at an individual level. Furthermore, providers would need to adjust to an environment in which a significant portion of their budget is not guaranteed but dependent on demand for their services. This transition has to be handled cautiously so as not to destabilise the market and leave individuals with fewer choices than before (Bennett, 2012).

The second, more significant, challenge is that many of the resources that could support PHBs are currently tied up in acute care settings. The PHB evaluation demonstrated that PHB holders made less use of inpatient, Accident and Emergency and GP services than those in the control group, saving £1,300 in inpatient costs per person per year (Forder et al, 2012). A report by the National Audit Office has criticised the NHS for its slowness in developing alternatives to hospital admission, citing the continuing increase in emergency admissions as a significant problem given current financial constraints (NAO, 2013). PHBs provide one such alternative. However, releasing funding from the acute sector to fund PHBs and shift the NHS towards a more preventative approach is a long-standing challenge (Purdy, 2010).

A larger, stronger evidence base will be required to convince decision makers to proceed with significant reconfiguration. Strategies have been outlined to enable commissioners to move away from block contracts and decommission existing services, for example the use of CQUIN targets, but most of this knowledge remains theoretical (Audit Commission, 2012b). More practical examples of how these strategies can be implemented will be necessary to give policymakers the confidence to strengthen existing commitments around PHBs for long-term conditions.

The challenge of clinical buy-in

Despite a three-year pilot, a national commitment to roll-out, inclusion in the NHS Mandate and the NHS Operating Framework, most clinicians, particularly doctors, are still relatively unaware of PHBs (BMA, 2012). Where they are aware, many remain sceptical despite support for the policy from the Royal College of GPs and Royal College of Psychiatrists (Mathers et al, 2012; ADASS and RCPsych, 2013). This is perhaps unsurprising given that PHBs are a fundamental challenge to the way in which most NHS clinicians are trained.

All of this is in sharp contrast to the traditional approach to clinical decision making – still prevalent in the NHS – in which clinicians are seen as the only competent decision makers, with an expectation that they will make decisions for rather than with patients (Coulter and Collins, 2011).

PHBs are rooted in a genuine partnership between the lived experience of individuals and families and the learned experience of clinical staff, tipping the current balance of power in the NHS more in favour of individuals and families (DH, 2012g). PHBs recognise that the day-to-day management of long-term conditions more often falls to individuals and families than clinical professionals and without fully understanding how a condition affects day-to-day life, treatment is less likely to be successful (Epstein et al, 2010).

If PHBs are to become part of the mainstream NHS, clinicians will need to see them as part of their toolkit to improve the health and wellbeing of those with long-term conditions alongside other shared decisions-making approaches such as Year of Care (Alakeson et al, 2013). Clinical resistance has not been absent in CHC. However, CHC has a clear advantage over other parts of the NHS and that is its relationship with social care. In many local areas, CHC teams have worked closely with local authority colleagues to implement PHBs, learning from and drawing on the experience of implementing personal budgets.

Building support for PHBs among clinicians outside of CHC will necessitate addressing two important barriers. The first is the apparent tension between evidence-based medicine and PHBs. PHBs are not restricted to interventions and treatments that are approved by the National Institute for Health and Care Excellence, which causes controversy (NMHDU, 2011). However, this fails to recognise the limitations of the current evidence base in knowing what will work for any one individual rather than at the population level and also in relation to wider health and wellbeing outcomes, such as remaining in employment. Here the current evidence base has little to offer (Alakeson and Perkins, 2012; Glasby et al, 2013). There are individuals with long-term conditions for whom the current set of evidence-based approaches do not work well (Mathers et al, 2012). They are repeat users of services and, for these individuals, PHBs offer clinicians an important tool with which to experiment and build a new, more personalised evidence base in partnership with individuals themselves.

The second important area of concern for clinicians is around risk and quality of care (Mathers et al, 2012). There are concerns about individuals putting themselves at risk by making different choices from the ones that clinicians would make on their behalf, as well as concerns about a deterioration in the quality of care if individuals go outside the boundaries of qualified providers, evidence-based care and accepted clinical approaches. This is despite strong evidence of the limitations of traditional approaches to quality assurance and safeguarding in the NHS (DH, 2012h; Francis, 2013). However, evidence to date and from social care suggests the opposite: individuals are less at risk if they are fully engaged in planning their care as an equal partner and can put in place contingencies (Health Foundation, 2010; Gadsby, 2013). Greater choice and control appear to improve perceived quality because care is better tailored to the needs and preferences of individuals.

Building bottom-up demand for PHBs

One of the drivers for the implementation of the national PHB pilot was the strong campaigning by parents of children who became eligible for CHC. Children and their families transitioning into adult services often found themselves in the position of qualifying for NHS care and as a result losing their ability to control their own care through a direct payment. Instead, they were offered a traditional care agency commissioned by the NHS (Alakeson, 2010). Having experienced choice and control in children's services, families saw no reason why they could not enjoy the same in the NHS and a small number of families secured the right to control their own services even before the pilot programme began (DH, 2010f).

However, this same level of bottom-up demand does not exist in the rest of the NHS. This is not to say that satisfaction is always high elsewhere. It is more that awareness of PHBs is low among individuals who use the NHS, as it is among clinicians. The large third sector organisations that might have been the natural allies of individuals were at the outset relatively cool towards PHBs (House of Commons, 2009). This has shifted over time as several organisations, for example Age UK and Rethink, have played a brokerage role as part of the pilot programme.

Aside from a lack of awareness, there is also a long-standing tendency for individuals to defer to clinicians, much as there is a tendency for clinicians to make decisions on behalf of their patients. As one GP in Kent put it:

> 'Doctors have too much knowledge and power and patients are too ready to defer to doctors because they believe they know everything. As a result, the conversation moves away too easily from how a patient wants to improve her life to medical complaints and clinical care.' (Alakeson, 2014, pp 98–99)

Paternalism has dominated the NHS and individuals will take time to adjust to a culture that demands more from them and expects them to take greater responsibility. But taking control brings benefits. The national evaluation found that improvements in wellbeing for PHB holders are closely linked to taking more control (Forder et al, 2012, p 79). Some people who are heavy users of the NHS can become so dependent on services that they lose the confidence to take control. Their identity becomes that of a patient or service user rather than the NHS enabling them to be a parent, employee or musician (Repper and Perkins, 2003). For these people, choice and control can feel daunting, particularly if they are not well supported to make choices and given time to expand their horizons. In this context, peer support can be a valuable tool to help individuals see new possibilities (Repper and Carter, 2010).

CCGs and clinicians may feel pressure from policymakers to implement PHBs. But to be a powerful engine for change, this needs to be combined with real demand from individuals. The Department of Health invested in the development of a national peer network to ensure that the voice of users was at the centre of the development of PHBs and peer networks are now being sustained and developed in some local areas. Other initiatives such as Peoplehub and Partners in Health also bring together PHB holders in order to influence developments, share information and build momentum behind roll-out. More activities such as these will be needed to change the culture of the NHS if PHBs are to spread more widely.

Maintaining the political consensus for PHBs

While PHBs will always remain a voluntary approach, there are benefits to the wider NHS if they can achieve a certain scale. If 10% of spending on long-term conditions were delivered through PHBs, this would no doubt force the rest of the system to also be more responsive to individuals. But getting from a few thousand budgets to a several hundred thousand will necessitate changing current approaches to commissioning, building support among clinicians and fostering stronger demand for PHBs from individuals and families. It will also critically depend on maintaining the cross-party consensus that has allowed PHBs to develop.

Each party may have a different reason for being in favour of PHBs but this has enabled a pilot started by the previous Labour government to be continued and extended by the coalition government, with clear support from both sides of the coalition being expressed at different times. Cross-party support allows investments to be made in service reconfiguration and in the painstaking work of culture change, safe in the knowledge that a change of government will not result in a change of policy direction. Addressing the challenges outlined above will be made significantly more difficult if there is a breakdown in this cross-party consensus.

For this reason, it is worrying to hear senior Labour and Conservative figures express reservations about PHBs (Johnson, 2013; Burton, 2013). Their critique is usually two-fold. The first is that PHBs and personal budgets drive fragmentation when the pressing need is for greater service integration. This is a familiar fault line but one that ignores the fact that integration is best achieved at the individual level – integrating services around the needs of a person not organisations. This requires access to different service options. Diversity of supply, therefore, becomes a precondition for integration, not a threat to it (Collins, 2012). Already there are several examples of successful integration around a person's needs through integrated personal health and social care budgets. The second is that a personalised NHS needs more than PHBs. This is undeniably the case and no one has ever claimed otherwise. A truly personalised NHS will need a range of tools that are relevant to different parts of the service. However, PHBs have an important part to play in supporting self-management for those with long- term conditions.

Whether it is high-speed rail or healthcare, investment in innovation will only be made if those who have to invest and make fundamental changes to the way in which they operate can have confidence in a stable policy environment. More than anything, this will be critical for the future of PHBs.

Part Five
Responses and conclusions

Advancing the positives of personalisation / person-centred support: a multi-perspective view

Peter Beresford

Introduction

We should not be surprised if the issue of personalisation and personal budgets has come to be seen as controversial and contentious. What perhaps would be more concerning would be if it were treated as straightforward and without complexity. Indeed, that has been one of the significant features of political approaches to personalisation. It has gained support from all three main political parties and tended to be treated as unproblematic. However, as soon as we consider the context of this idea and development, it becomes possible to see some of the serious traps lying in wait for it, and also to begin to explore ways of overcoming them.

First, a point about my position on this issue. Historically, there has been some polarisation of discussion, with some people and constituencies strongly for or strongly against personalisation and personal budgets. This has at times been a fraught and disturbing situation, with some commentators who have been critical of this development marginalised and excluded (Boxall et al, 2009). My background as a long-term health and social care service user has put me in a different position. Over the years since the 1970s, a number of different developments have taken place in social care (extending in some cases to health). These include the establishment of social services departments, the introduction of community social work and then community care, care management, the 'purchaser–provider split' and now 'personalisation'. Each of these innovations has been heralded as offering more cost–effective and responsive services and systems of support. In some cases, the rhetoric of increased choice and control that has come to be associated with personalisation has also been emphasised – notably in the case of community care. The evidence has indicated that each of these developments, some of which like community social work have been effectively short-lived, has failed to bring the gains promised for them. It is not necessarily clear whether this is because of limitations of their own, or because of the chronic underfunding and other problems that have affected social care and the particular way in which they were implemented. When adult service users are asked about their experience of social care, they tend to present an overall picture of provision that is inadequate in scale and quality, with diminishing access and availability.

Service user perspectives

Understandably, service users tend to be less interested in the supposed or intended goals and principles of policy and services than in what services are actually like as they experience them, and the resulting picture has long been a discouraging one (Harding and Beresford, 1996; Beresford, 2007; Beresford and Andrews, 2012). Because of this, a focus on the day-to-day reality of provision has tended to be my starting point for considering policy and practice developments. It seems helpful to focus less on the rationales that are attached to them by policymakers and their proponents and more on what actual positive difference they make for people, how widespread and inclusive they are, and whether they are sustainable. The principles associated with personalisation and personal budgets, generally presented as enabling greater choice and control, rather like sentiments in favour of 'mom and apple pie', have always been of the vague and feel-good kind that would be very difficult to disagree with.

My involvement in the psychiatric system survivor movement began in 1987, after in-patient hospital experience, getting involved in user-led organisations like Survivors Speak Out and Mind Link (Beresford, 2010). I also developed links with disability activists and disabled people's organisations. This was at the time when such organisations and individuals were pioneering new forms of collective support provision and also 'direct payments', a new idea from the disabled people's movement based on the social model of disability and the associated philosophy of independent living (Morris, 1993). At the heart of these ideas was the belief that disabled people should have the support they needed and access to mainstream life and services to enable them to live their lives on as equal terms as possible as non-service users. These ideas were widely discussed, had a large impact on many disabled people and their lives and influenced disability discourse and policy both in the UK and internationally (Brissenden, 1986; Morris,

1993; Oliver, 1996). In the UK, they notably led to the passing of the 1996 Community Care (Direct Payments) Act, which came into force in 1997, and the 2008 Independent Living Strategy, which officially endorsed the philosophy of the disabled people's independent living movement and promoted the establishment of a national network of disabled people's/service user-led organisations (ODI, 2008). These developments were the context for and antecedents of subsequent calls for personal, or, as they were also then called, 'individual' budgets by organisations like In Control, Demos and the National Institute for Mental Health in England (NIMHE). However, as noted in Chapter Two and as I stated at the time on numerous conference platforms, this historic debt tended not to be acknowledged.

The circumstances of social care

This brings us back to the difficulties and contentiousness that have surrounded personal budgets and personalisation, since these jargonistic terms first came into policy use in the early 21st century. Although personalisation's advocates have made the case for it across a wide range of social policies, including housing, health and education, its developments has been most closely associated with social care, one of the most under-developed and under-financed areas of UK social policy. While in many other European countries health and social care have developed together essentially as one policy, in the UK, particularly in England, since the creation of the post-war welfare state, there has been a growing separation between the two and they have become increasing separate policies, differently funded, differently organised and coming under different control. This has not only been damaging and difficult for each policy, but has also created many problems for service users trying to negotiate their way between them and put barriers in the way of their successful reunification and integration.

While the National Health Service is prized by the public and has become a totem of public opinion no political party wants to be seen as putting at risk, the same has not been true of local government-led social care. This is not well name-checked by the public who are largely unfamiliar with the term, does not carry the same political clout as the NHS (despite the lack of logic in this) and also – as we have seen, during the coalition government's imposition of public service cuts in the name of 'austerity' – has minimal protection from draconian reductions in public spending.

Between 2012 and 2013, some major concerns were highlighted about social care. These include:

- the routine use and expansion of a culture of zero-hours contracts for face-to-face social care staff required to undertake the most sensitive, intimate and personal tasks in people's homes;
- social care workers' pay and conditions being often inferior to even the most basic mainstream employment, with individuals frequently having to work at rates of pay below the minimum wage as they are not paid for travel, and if provided at all, training and supervision sometimes taking place in workers' own time;
- the widespread use of 15-minute time slots for providing domiciliary care, so that for adequate time to be available for service users, workers may be forced to work longer hours unpaid;
- a trend towards an increasing amount of social care provision coming under the control of large for-profit companies, including private equity companies, that are minimally accountable and have minimal transparency;
- the UK's biggest care home provider, Southern Cross, going out of business without proper alternatives in place for its 30,000 older residential service users;
- appalling cases of abuse and neglect, for example, in provision for people with learning difficulties at Winterbourne View, Bristol and at Orchid View residential home in West Sussex for older people where five residents died;
- serious concerns relating to the regulator, the Care Quality Commission;
- eligibility to social care through Fair Access to Care Services (FACS) criteria becoming increasingly limited, undermining any aspirations to prevention; and
- financial allocations and their equivalent to individuals being reduced in line with funding cuts.

Social care is clearly a policy in a state of crisis and disarray. Government proposals for reform are themselves limited and indeed, in relation to funding reform, fall short even of the modest proposals offered by the Dilnot Commission, which came in for major criticism from the private sector, the Association of Directors of Adult Social Services and service users and carers (Beresford, 2011a, 2011b). To add to this, disabled people and other groups of social care service users seem to be bearing the brunt of the damaging effects resulting from the coalition's radical welfare reforms, which are taking billions from their incomes, while doing little to offer meaningful alternative opportunities in employment (Davison and Rutherford, 2012). Meanwhile, the Secretary of State for Health, Jeremy Hunt, used the 2013 National Children and Adult

Services Conference, the premier social care event in the calendar, to impute blame to the families of 'as many as 800,000 chronically lonely older people' and to contrast this with the 'reverence and respect for older people in Asian culture' (BBC, 2013).

Personal budgets in perspective

Think Local, Act Personal (TLAP) is the 'national, cross sector leadership partnership focused on driving forward work with personalisation'.[1] It has a board of 17 members, one of whom is a service user/disabled person. There are no members from disabled people's or user-led organisations. TLAP is committed to the goals of people having 'better lives through more choice and control over the support they use: often referred to as "personalisation" '.[2] This reflects and reiterates the dominant discourse around personalisation. This has, as we have seen, been framed in very general terms of increasing choice and control. Originally, the government framed this as being achieved by making an offer of personal budgets and then subsequently talked about personalisation in more general terms as a goal for all social care provision, both residential and domiciliary. So personalisation has appeared to be both means (personal budgets) and end (choice and control).

It has therefore always seemed important to me to gain as good an understanding as possible *from the evidence* of what personal budgets were actually achieving and also how best to advance the broader goal of personalisation. It is these two issues, particularly the latter, that I am concerned with addressing in this overview chapter.

Chapter Two of this volume explored independent evidence highlighting some of the problems with personal budgets. This data can now be updated with more research, in which I have been involved (Slasberg, et al, 2013). One additional point should be made about evidence in relation to personal budgets and personalisation. The generally accepted standard for rigour, reliability and independence in research is that publications are subjected to a recognised process of peer review. Very little of the evidence that has been central in the advancement of personal budgets policy has been peer reviewed in this way. Instead it has tended to come from individual case examples, statements, articles and research reports, often from organisations closely linked with personal budgets whose interests lie in their advancement. Other independent evidence, for example, that regularly produced by Community Care, has tended to paint a much more critical picture of personal budgets. The evidence offered now has been through such a process of peer review as discussed above. Key findings from this latest research with data from 2011-12 indicate the following:

- There is no relationship between the up-front 'indicative' allocations of personal budgets and what people actually get (from freedom of information requests to nearly a third of all councils). The average difference between the two is between two- and three-fold. As a result, up-front allocation, key to the dominant model of personal budgets, is all but meaningless.
- Nonetheless, a major new bureaucracy has been generated to ensure the delivery of this process, the resource allocation system (RAS). This is evidenced in reports by practitioners, and evidence of a major loss of productivity in fieldwork, perhaps worth as much as £0.5 billion a year. Central government demands councils deliver up-front allocations as the performance measure of delivery of personalisation.
- There is no relationship between the number of people said to have a personal budget and the number of service users who report themselves as having control over their lives, which was one of the central promises of the strategy.
- A belief that the personal budget strategy is working is being maintained through the selective and misleading use of data. This includes 'packing' survey samples with people who use a direct payment and who tend to receive a higher proportion of funding. Direct payments have been enabling people to have better outcomes for many years and have no need of the additional provision – the up-front allocation – of the personal budget strategy to continue to do so (Slasberg et al, 2013).

The government is additionally committed to introducing personal health budgets (PHBs) in the NHS from 2014. All people with Continuing Healthcare needs will have a right to a personal health budget, while local commissioning groups will be enabled to offer them to others with a long-term condition. A report on a three-year programme of PHB pilots, commissioned by the Department of Health, concluded that they have improved outcomes and are generally cost-effective (Forder et al, 2012). The government is attributing these improved outcomes from the pilots to a process similar to the one introduced in social care, called self-directed support – which, as we have seen, is based on the individual being given a sum of money 'up front' with which to plan their own support. Yet a review of the evidence suggests that this is not an accurate analysis of the findings it commissioned. The authors of this evaluation concluded that what was important was not having an 'up-front allocation', but that 'personal health budgets should be configured to give recipients choice and flexibility over how the budget can be used' (Forder et al, 2012, p 158). This is exactly what might be expected; that where service users get the support that matches their unique needs, they are likely to have better outcomes. Thus, up-front allocation was not related to better outcomes. This also, of course, leaves unresolved issues of ensuring that resource levels are sufficient to achieve this, and to achieve it in line with the NHS's fundamental universalist principles, for all patients/ service users (Slasberg et al, 2014).

At this point, it may be helpful to review this discussion of the official/ dominant discourse about personalisation and personal budgets so far. These terms have sometimes been used by government and others interchangeably. Sometimes they have been presented as both a means and an end, and sometimes the two appear to have been confused. Personal budgets were offered as a cheaper and more effective route to greater user choice and control. In the event, what was presented as a solution has been shown to bring significant problems of its own. A key point for me is how could personal budgets on their own ever have been expected to offer a solution to the much broader problems associated with social care? As Melanie Henwood argues in Chapter Eight, if giving people money to get the support they want would solve the problem, why is it that so many self-funders, including those who are better off, have ended up institutionalised, when theoretically many could have the real choice that is supposed to be available to the individual consumer?

Personalisation in context

It was because the whole logic of personal budgets seemed inherently inadequate that a consortium of us responded to and successfully bid for a call from the Joseph Rowntree Foundation to undertake a major UK-wide research and development project, 'The Standards We Expect', whose focus was personalisation, or as we described it, to avoid jargon, person-centred support (Beresford et al, 2011). The key aims of the project were to find out what person-centred support/ personalisation meant to people, what barriers they saw in its way and how these might be overcome. We wanted to explore, rather than take as given, some of the key issues and concepts that seemed to be associated with personalisation and personal budgets. So the first question to be addressed, rather than accepting or imposing a definition, was what was meant by the term.

There is a key point that needs to be made here. As has been said, direct payments were an idea and initiative that grew out of the disabled people's movement. However, personal budgets, despite being strongly indebted to direct payments, were not led by disabled people or other service users. Key organisations involved, including In Control, NIMHE and TLAP, were not user-led. Key individuals involved were not disabled people or service users, but rather professionally qualified and networked 'experts' and consultants. The support of service users and their organisations was enlisted and service-user stories were important in the selling of personal budgets. But this was not a service user-led development. The move from disabled people's direct payments to what became government personal budgets policy was associated with a radical shift in control. It was also associated with a significant shift in ideology. The direct payments developed by the disabled people's movement were liberatory in intent and were coupled to values of empowerment. Retrospectively Simon Duffy said that a fair allocation for a personal budget was 'enough money to enable independent living and full citizenship' (Duffy, 2012b). This is in line with disabled people's philosophy of independent living. But in 2006, when Duffy and In Control were selling personal budgets to the government, they described the resource allocation system as one 'designed to offer openly, publicly and fairly an allocation of funding that was affordable within current authority budgets' (Poll et al, 2006). This is something very different – personal budgets based not on need but on funding levels acknowledged to be inadequate.

For this reason, we were especially anxious that the Standards We Expect project should involve the key perspectives concerned with person-centred support/personalisation and that it should be a participatory project. We identified these key perspectives as those of service users, face-to-face practitioners and carers. The Standards We Expect consortium involved four organisations: Shaping Our Lives (a user-led organisation, which led the project); Values Into Action (a voluntary organisation where people with learning difficulties and non-disabled people worked together on equal terms); the Centre for Social Action, de Montfort University; and the Centre for Citizen Participation, Brunel University. It was made up of service users, researchers and practitioners and ran over four years. It worked in eight sites with a broader network of 12 organisations and services, involving more than 350 service users. It included a very wide range of service users in a diverse range of social care, health and housing settings, providing a variety of support services, both urban and rural. It worked in a participatory way, adopting user-controlled research principles, emphasising the involvement of service users, face-to-face practitioners and carers, and exploring their ideas and experience about person-centred support. It offered participants a range of support for taking person-centred support forward in their localities, including information and guidance, collective forums, capacity building and opportunities for shared learning.

Research findings for key questions

The project focused on three particular questions. These were:

- What does person-centred support/personalisation mean to you?
- What barriers do you see in the way of person-centred support/ personalisation?
- How do you think these barriers can be overcome?

What person-centred support/personalisation means

While there were some variations in emphasis, significantly, the meanings service users, practitioners and carers attached to personalisation were very similar. Thus, a consensus definition emerged from the project, one that was consistent both with ideas of 'person-centred planning' and 'independent living'. Both of these were concerned with putting in place the support people needed to live their lives on as equal terms as possible with non-service users, rather than seeing service users as needing 'care' because of perceived deficits and pathologies (Beresford et al, 2011, pp 39-46).

Participants' definition of person-centred support was strongly based on values rather than techniques or procedures. Key components cited were:

- putting the person at the centre, rather than fitting them into services;
- treating service users as individuals;
- ensuring choice and control for service users;
- setting goals with service users for support;
- emphasising the importance of the relationship between service users and practitioners;
- listening to service users and acting on what they say;
- providing up-to-date, accessible information about appropriate services;
- flexibility; and

- a positive approach, which highlights what service users might be able to do, not what they cannot do (Beresford et al, 2011, pp 46-63).

Participants spelt out what they meant by this:

'... at the weekends you might want to have a lie in because you have been out clubbing Friday night and you might want to not have anyone interfering and coming in until midday maybe to support you if you need it.' (Service user)

'It's about being organic, that's reacting to individuals. So that's about being person-centred, listening to people and what they want and providing those services which cut into the finances rather than providing what we've been dictated to provide or what we think is right or what would be a good idea, "or that would be nice, wouldn't it". Just encouraging your staff to think like that, that's what we've done.' (Practitioner)

'It's starting with the person around what that particular person's needs are and matching the services with their needs rather than the other way round.' (Practitioner)

'Giving me choice and control, putting me first.' (Service user)

'Having control so that when things aren't working for you, you can say so.' (Service user)

'It's about fitting the services around people rather than people into the services.' (Manager)

Barriers in the way of person-centred support

Participants in the project highlighted a range of major barriers that they felt undermined person-centred support and restricted their rights. Not only did each of these create its own obstacles inhibiting such an approach, but combined they magnified such difficulties. Key barriers identified included:

- the lack of a well-supported, skilled and well-trained workforce and low levels of staffing. Generally, poor terms and conditions were associated with low retention and high turnover rates, offering little prospect of ensuring an adequate workforce to match predictions of greatly increasing demand;

- increasing reliance being placed on family members as 'informal carers'. Without sufficient support for carers themselves, or help for them to facilitate service users' independence, there is an inadequate and inappropriate basis for meeting increased future need;

- the lives of many long-term and residential service users being restricted by continuing institutionalisation. This disempowers them, undermines their confidence, limits their potential and prevents them gaining the skills to live fuller, more equal lives;

- organisational barriers to person-centred support. These operate at all levels. Participants cited increased bureaucratisation, tightening administrative controls, inflexible organisations, crude target setting and an emphasis on 'negative risk', often framed in terms of health and safety requirements;

- social care practice. Participants saw this as following from a disempowering service culture that is still often paternalistic and inflexible – 'making unhelpful assumptions about what service users can and can't do', as one said – and restricting the crucial relationship between them and practitioners;

- service users' restricted access to mainstream policies and services, keeping them within social care services and undermining the holistic approach of person-centred support to live on as equal and inclusive terms as non-service users as possible. Three particular areas mentioned were travel and transport, education and continuing disability discrimination. People living in rural areas and from black and minority ethnic communities faced additional barriers;

- barriers relating to service users' circumstances and experience. Many lacked the support they needed to be able to access and take advantage of person-centred support. There is a lack of capacity building through ensuring accessible information, advice, guidance and advocacy (Beresford et al, 2011, pp 99-256).

Participants' comments gave flesh-and-blood reality to these issues.

> 'The staff aren't well trained; if you know what goes on in a person with dementia's mind then you have more patience and understand. But if you don't have any training, then you aren't going to know, so it makes it difficult.' (Practitioner)

'Your parents are a massive thing but they need to know that, yeah they can care for you, and yeah they can do what they like for you, but they need to know that you want your space.' (Service user)

'We are not allowed to talk to people on the other table. We wait for staff to finish their tea. When staff get up they say what people are on the rota to do. You can't get up until the staff say so.' (Service user)

'You're going to the supermarket to do your shopping and it's something that everyone in the world does and you have to do a risk assessment on it!' (Practitioner)

'I think people will come and ask you what you want, but you don't necessarily always know what is available to ask for! So there will always be somebody who will ask, but you won't necessarily know what there is to ask for.' (Service user)

'Their human rights are not being met. Not only by the government – local councils, local traders. Last night we wanted to go out for a meal. Three restaurants we tried to get into. We had two disabled people with motorised chairs, two [non-disabled] people among us. Three restaurants, no ramps, no lifts, no nothing.' (Carer/relative)

Overcoming barriers

We found much being done in local areas and services to overcome these barriers, despite the constraints at work on managers, practitioners, service users and carers. The development phase of the project, where the project team worked in the different sites to support more person-centred support/personalisation, also highlighted ways of challenging existing difficulties.

The project also found that all the efforts on the ground to challenge barriers were not enough to enable person-centred support to become the norm for all service users. Barriers seemed to be rooted in two major problems: the chronic inadequacy of social care funding and the continued existence of a social care culture at odds with person-centred support. This problematic culture was reflected in continuing institutionalisation, control, paternalism and inflexibility in services and reliance on a 'deficit' model rather than on the philosophy of independent living as the basis for providing support. Funding problems also seemed to lie at the heart of workforce inadequacies, over-reliance on unpaid carers, insufficient and inaccessible mainstream services and lack of suitable advocacy, advice and information services. These two overarching barriers – of inadequate funding and inappropriate culture – also seemed to work in complex and damaging interrelation with each other and were not amenable to isolated action at local level but instead demanded strategic policy change from central government

Conclusion

We concluded from these findings that efforts to move to person-centred support/personalisation were being undermined by social care's funding problems. It was difficult to see from the project how meaningful personalisation could be rolled out and achieved for all on a sustainable basis for the future, without social care being securely and adequately funded. The conclusion from the findings was that funding through general taxation was likely to be the most viable and effective way of achieving this. The unification of NHS and social care funding arrangements also seemed likely to help overcome arbitrary and unhelpful divisions between the two services. We also concluded that to achieve the radical changes that were required would require concerted policy change that combined top-down and bottom-up approaches and was committed to a participatory approach to reform (Beresford et al, 2011, pp 253-90).

In the light of the findings from this project, personal budgets policy seems even more like a chimera. It hardly seems surprising if efforts to achieve radical change in social care through their isolated implementation, based on neoliberal government ideology at a time of draconian public spending cuts, appear to be failing. Personal budgets have conspicuously failed to 'transform' social care as government and its advocates claimed they would. All the key problems of workforce, inadequate market and so on continue. How could it ever be expected that on their own they could make any major positive difference, least of all to the lives of most social care service users? Furthermore, personalised support sadly remains as far, if not further away, from being achieved. Structural developments in social care, including the increasing and damaging role of large for-profit organisations, appear instead to be working in a different direction.

Doubtless direct payments provided in the flexible and supported way originally envisaged by the disabled people's movement, in line with its philosophy of independent living and operating with the support of a national network of user-led organisations, could have a valuable contribution to make to the achievement of personalised social care and health for many more. But this would demand a real political commitment to social care, its re-prioritisation and urgent new public investment, none of which appear likely in the short term, even if ultimately there may be no alternative. The personal budgets story so far, especially from the perspective of most of those in need of social care support, tends to reinforce long-standing lessons from general human experience, from politics to ebay, that if it looks like a rip off it probably is. If the claims that are made for a service or product seem too good to be true, in all likelihood they are.

Notes

[1] See www.thinklocalactpersonal.org.uk/About_us/

[2] See www.thinklocalactpersonal.org.uk/Browse/ThinkLocalActPersonal/

EIGHTEEN

After personalisation

Simon Duffy

Every idea can be interpreted in different ways, but some ideas are more open to interpretation than others. Personalisation is particularly open-ended. Opinion differs about its authors, its purpose, its content, its impact and its real meaning.

In this chapter, I am going to write as one of those associated with its development. I will describe my own thinking, what happened as my ideas were put into practice and how those ideas were absorbed into the broader concept of personalisation. I will then try to draw some lessons about the challenges ahead.

This will not be an objective account of personalisation. It is an insider's account of personalisation, with all the loss of perspective that guarantees. The one advantage of my account will be to reveal those parts of the development of personalisation that are hidden to the disengaged observer.

Citizenship and community

One of the most common criticisms of personalisation is that it is a right-wing idea (Ferguson, 2007). This is a curious criticism, because it seems to imply that there is something right-wing about wanting to improve the legal and economic power of disabled people. But it is such a persistent criticism that it cannot simply be dismissed. And it is certainly true that some advocates of personalisation have seen it as a new kind of consumerism (Bartlett, 2009).

Personally, I do not think the left–right continuum is the only or the most useful way of thinking about public policy. In fact, the experience of disabled people provides powerful testimony for a different way of thinking (Duffy, 2010). Two ideas in particular seem to be missing from the simplified left–right battle:

- citizenship – that we should live, in all our diversity, as free and equal citizens; and

- community – that we should live together with a shared commitment to the world.

This different way of thinking offers a better way of understanding the lessons learned by disabled people over the past 200 years. For disabled people did not find that they were liberated by markets during the growth of industrialisation and the philosophy of liberalism in the 19th century. In fact, this period marked the birth of the large-scale institution, designed to swallow thousands of disabled people and keep them away from community.

Even worse, eugenics, a philosophy that was born out of Darwinism, proposed that some human lives were worth much less than others, and so institutions were used to segregate and sterilise disabled people, particularly in the first half of the 20th century. Hitler's Germany took this thinking to its logical extreme and disabled people became the first victims of the Holocaust, and about 250,000 disabled people were murdered (Evans, 2004).

After World War II there was a greater emphasis on human rights and, at least publicly, eugenics was disgraced (Duffy, 2013a). However, institutions continued to flourish. The peak population for institutions in the UK was in the 1970s, and institutions continued to grow in the latter part of the 20th century, across the developed world. But disabled people also learned that, while markets did not protect them, neither did the state. The state simply absorbed and supported those institutions – employing the doctors, nurses or other staff who ran them.

When the institutions did begin to close, it was not just because the state had woken up to how terrible they were. It was because disabled people, families, ordinary citizens and enlightened professionals began to create alternative forms of support and to challenge the state-run system. The idea that institutions were shut because of right-wing ideology is nonsense, but it is interesting to note that left-wing governments were certainly not always alive to the rights of disabled people; often the interests of state employees and unionised professionals ranked higher.

The citizenship perspective offers a distinct critique of modern society; however, the voices of disabled people and their perspective rarely touch the mainstream media, or even mainstream academic thinking about the welfare system. References to disability within the main texts on political theory or economics are very scarce and when they do occur they are more likely to reveal a paternalistic attitude than any real understanding of the real and equal value of all disabled people (Rawls, 1971).

Self-directed support

Certainly, disability did not feature in my own life or in my academic training. It was only in 1988, when working as a junior NHS manager, that I discovered that people with learning disabilities existed and that they had been condemned, for decades, to live in inhuman institutions. That discovery has remained the inspiration for my own work for more than 20 years.

In 1990 I got a secondment from NHS management to work in a community organisation providing support and housing to people who had returned to London from long-stay institutions. I found these community care services an improvement on the institutions, but far from ideal. The move to community care was rarely a move to citizenship or inclusion in community. Instead, people found themselves living in group homes, attending day centres and using special buses. The old institution had been replaced with a new institution – made up of segregated services, controlled by professionals and accountable to government – not to people themselves.

This was all the more paradoxical because the rhetoric of community care, and the philosophies and theories that inspired it, were so positive and interesting (Towell, 1988). Ideas like the social model of disability, normalisation, social role valorisation or inclusion were widespread. But there was a huge gulf between the rhetoric and the reality.

There were many reasons for this gulf and for the poor quality of so many community care services and as I worked to provide better support to people I learned a great deal from others who had been struggling with the same issues. In particular, I found that champions of inclusion, like John O'Brien and Beth Mount, had already demonstrated that better lives are not created by means of services; instead, people must build better lives for themselves, in partnership with family and community, and around their own values, needs and aspirations. This seemed to me to offer a much more powerful way of thinking and my experience of working with people and families reinforced the logic of this approach; respecting people and their communities really works.

However, this raised interesting questions about how services should be organised (Duffy, 1996). As it stands, the system works to the Professional Gift Model: tax-funded services are designed by professionals and given to individuals, and the individual's power to control and redefine these services is minimal (Figure 18.1). This is not a minor issue. If you live in a care home or attend a day centre, almost every aspect of your life is outside your control.

Figure 18.1: Professional Gift versus Citizenship Models of support

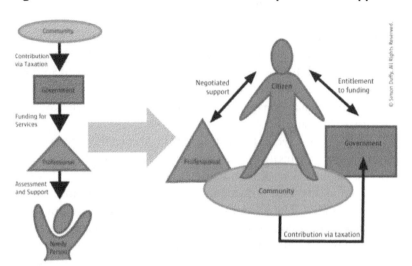

So a different model seemed necessary. I called this model the Citizenship Model, and this model works in a different way:

- Funding is individualised – you can shape support to suit your needs.
- Funding is an entitlement – it is yours by right and others cannot dictate to you how you must live.
- Funding is flexible – it can be used however best strengthens your community life.

Not only is it possible to imagine a different approach, it is even possible to make changes within the current system that mimic the Citizenship Model, rather than the Professional Gift Model. My work over the next 12 years, from 1990 to 2002, focused primarily on testing and developing different way of bringing the Citizenship Model to life:

- 1990–94: early experiments in individualised funding and services in Southwark, south London, around individuals who did not want to live in group homes but who wanted homes of their own (Duffy, 1992);
- 1996–99: the founding of Inclusion Glasgow (and other organisations in Scotland) to provide flexible personalised support using individual service funds to help people leave institutions and establish their own lives (Fitzpatrick, 2010);
- 1999–2002: early trials of self-directed support in North Lanarkshire and East Renfrewshire Council, using individual budgets to change

how the care management system worked and to increase people's capacity to make their own plans (Duffy and Sanderson, 2005).

Of course, these small-scale innovations were also happening in a much wider context (Glasby and Littlechild, 2009). In 1988, the Independent Living Fund enabled some disabled people to take control of their own support and in 1996 the Direct Payments Act give disabled people the right to convert their social care support into cash. There has also been a number of important experiments in individualised funding in Canada, the US and New Zealand. Individualised funding was also fundamental to many Scandinavian funding systems (Race, 2007).

From the successes and failures of my own work and the international evidence, I made a number of assumptions about the best design for self-directed support. Each of these assumptions is controversial, but much of what was original and innovative in the English experience of self-directed support is based on these assumptions. For better or worse, no other country had tried to develop self-directed support in quite this way before.

First, there was the up-front budget – what has become known as the individual or personal budget – and the use of the resource allocation system. The old system tended to place people in pre-purchased services (Duffy, 2005). Even when individual funding was used, it tended to be the professionals who would design the package of support, and then use this package to define the relevant budget (Figure 18.2). My own experience in the 1990s had persuaded me that up-front budgeting, where possible, was more empowering and increased:

- Creativity – when people know that they have a flexible budget, they can develop more creative solutions, building on their own resources and better linked to their own community.
- Responsibility – when people have a budget that is a clear entitlement and is protected for their benefit, they and those around them take more care to manage it effectively.
- Sustainability – when the system can set budgets based on its current expenditure, it is more willing to give away control, increase flexibility and let others get involved.

Second, there was the issue of brokerage. Early advocates of individual funding were convinced that independent professional support to make decisions was critical to helping people make good use of their own budget. My own experience of developing and using brokerage had

Figure 18.2: The shift to up-front budgeting and individual budgets

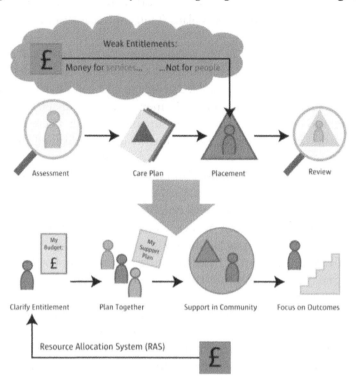

persuaded me of the opposite assumption (Duffy and Fulton, 2009). It seemed to me that a reliance on independent brokerage risked creating:

- dependency – many people, families and peers needed no or only minimal support to develop high-quality support for themselves or those they cared about;
- professionalisation – there was no need for yet another group of professionals to populate the lives of disabled people and their families;
- resistance – it is better to build on the best professional and community sources of expertise rather than try to replace them with a new kind of professional.

This is a particularly critical question for social workers, who can find their role being undermined by advocates of individualised funding who assume that they are either incompetent at offering good advice or that their role in setting budgets conflicts with their role as planners (Figure 18.3) (Duffy and Fulton, 2010). Obviously, the idea of up-front

Figure 18.3: Community brokerage

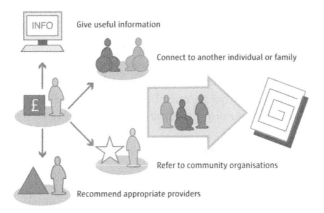

budgeting also changes things somewhat. If a budget can be outlined, without predefining the support package, there is less conflict for a social worker in being involved in planning.

The third design assumption was that every possible form of budget management should be open to disabled people and families. Legally, direct payments had opened up a vital alternative to the old system, enabling disabled people to manage their own budgets. But, so it seemed to me, there was also a role for other options: representatives managing budgets, trusts, services or independent agencies (Duffy, 2004).

It was these three design assumptions that I built into the first models of self-directed support, first in Scotland, and then later at In Control (Duffy, 2006). And this model of self-directed support had one further advantage – it meant that local authorities could experiment with this model of self-directed support quickly and with no additional costs. Budgets could be set within the framework of existing costs, no expensive systems of brokerage were required and it would be possible to work with people, families, providers and social workers to manage funds. By ruling no options out, but introducing a new level of transparency with different degrees of control, it seemed possible to move quickly to radical systemic change.

Of course, I had learned already that having an idea and making that idea real are two entirely different things. The real challenge was not just to create a new model of self-directed support, but also to get people to adopt, improve and develop that model.

The phases of personalisation

It is important to note that the term 'personalisation' was not used by those of us who were developing and implementing these new models of service delivery. Widespread use of the term only came later and played its own interesting role in how these ideas were implemented (Leadbeater et al, 2008). So we must begin before personalisation and for me that means beginning with self-directed support.

Realising self-directed support

In 2003, several local authorities had begun to work on the small-scale project that would become known as In Control. The initial goal was modest – to test self-directed support for small numbers of people, generally with complex learning disabilities. Using the model described earlier, a handful of local authorities were supported to create the systems necessary to make self-directed a reality. This meant:

- systems to set budgets;
- systems to help people plan;
- changes to how social workers (care managers) would work;
- changes in local rules and systems.

These changes were not easy, but when a small number of local authorities were found who were willing to work differently, it was possible to bring about quite radical changes – inside the older 'unreformed' system. This required an innovative space to be created, within the existing organisation, where new ways of working could be made possible.

In addition, In Control developed an interesting methodology for supporting local authorities and sharing these innovations more widely. One of my colleagues, Carl Poll, proposed that we use social marketing techniques:

- to create a distinct brand for In Control, including a memorable name (the name I had been using was the much less imaginative National Self-directed Support Programme);
- to publish accessible, easy-to-read information that could be used by anyone;
- to use a website to host the best tools and resources so that pilot sites could share information quickly and effectively;

- to build partnerships that let others share and use our ideas, for no fee.

In retrospect, this social marketing approach was critical to the early successes of In Control. The organisation was tiny and existed on minimal funding. But it was able to get its message across and build a wider movement precisely because it did not threaten others – it just offered a different path. However, the most important feature of these innovations was that they worked. People saw dramatic improvements in their lives, while also seeing costs reduce (Poll et al, 2006).

At the same time, during 2004, there was a growing awareness by some in the Labour government that this pilot presented them with an interesting policy success. A minister visited one of our pilot sites, I wrote a paper for the Cabinet Office, and there were a number of meetings and presentations for civil servants and others (Duffy, 2005a; 2005b). By the beginning of 2005, it appeared that the idea of self-directed support had finally arrived.

The battle for evidence

One of the most important lessons for all innovators in public policy is that there is no copyright on ideas. This means that you can have an idea, but you do not own it, and, once an idea is being used by powerful individuals and organisations, that idea is very likely to be used for very different purposes from those you might have intended.

One sign that this had already happened was that the term 'self-directed support' was not picked up by government; instead, it focused on the term 'individual budget'. In May 2005, the New Labour government, having made a manifesto commitment to give individual budgets to all older people, launched its Individual Budget Pilot Programme (IBPP). To an outsider, the idea of the IBPP will seem appropriate and rational. It was a multimillion pound randomised control trial that aimed to ascertain whether individual budgets were really effective. To an insider, the design, development and organisation of this pilot programme was curiously perverse:

- There would be 13 pilot sites, and three different universities involved in the research.
- Each pilot site could develop its own system of individual budgets.
- All the data from the pilot sites would be merged.

- Not only would local authorities be asked to set budgets from their own funding, but they would also be expected to somehow merge five other streams of funding controlled by Whitehall.
- In Control was to be excluded from the programme, as it would naturally be biased to its own models.
- In Control was no longer allowed to use the term 'individual budget' as it was now a government concept.

It was hard to see how any of this would work well. However, it set up an interesting new phase of development. While the government continued with the IBPP, In Control was allowed to work in parallel with other local authorities. As we could no longer use the term 'individual budget', we had to go through all our documentation and replace the word 'individual' with the word 'personal'.

Building on earlier work to develop the In Control brand, it was possible to enrol local authorities up and down the country to join In Control as members. Several authorities also agreed to be 'total transformation' sites, aiming to redesign their whole systems to use self-directed support for everyone. We also wrote, lobbied and spoke on platforms up and down England.

In less than two years, In Control had over 100 local authorities as members, thousands of people with individual budgets and further data showing improved outcomes and reduced costs (Poll and Duffy, 2008). What is more, the Association of Directors of Adult Social Services and the Minister for Social Care, Ivan Lewis, had become supportive of a change in policy.

The launch of personalisation

The key moment came in December 2007 when Ivan Lewis, backed by several government ministers, launched *Putting People First* (DH, 2007). This policy set out the government's vision for radical reform across adult social care and marked the beginning of what is now called personalisation. The ideas have now spread into children services, education and the NHS (Alakeson and Duffy, 2011).

It may be hard to appreciate what a radical change this new policy represented. Previous to this, the official policy of the Department of Health was that improvement and efficiency would come through bigger block contracts, regional commissioning policies and greater regulation. The idea that transferring more power to people was the key to positive change had seemed laughable. Yet *Putting People First* also represented the end of In Control's real influence. The document put the matter clearly:

> We recognise that organisations such as In Control, other voluntary organisations and some local authorities have been at the cutting edge of innovation in adult social care for some time. The Individual Budget, Partnerships for Older People and LinkAge Plus pilots have begun to demonstrate what works as well as identifying barriers to progress.
>
> However, national and local leadership is now essential if we are to achieve system-wide transformation. This is necessary because of demographic realities, but driven by a shared commitment to social justice. (DH, 2007, p 5)

Again the use of the term 'personalisation' signalled a change in emphasis. This term had been championed by Charles Leadbeater and Demos (Leadbeater et al, 2008). He argued that we had been previously been through an era of privatisation, but we were now to go through an era of personalisation. Public services would have to adapt and must offer tailored support. Self-directed support was, for him, one interesting example of this wider concept of personalisation.

The widening of the idea was combined with an enormous injection of extra spending. Consultancy organisations and think tanks suddenly became experts in personalisation, universities started talking about personalisation and local authorities began to create new posts for people to take a lead in personalisation. The government set about spending half a billion pounds on ideas that had, until that point, been developed almost for free.

Sadly, spending money in this way seems to have had the opposite impact to the one desired. When there is too much money, there is no incentive to:

- learn from your colleagues or those who've already made good progress;
- minimise costs and get rid of old systems that are not working; or
- trust people and empower frontline staff.

Paradoxically, the new personalisation programme seemed to lead to no new ideas or practical innovations. Instead, money was wasted and old ideas were recycled rather than improved. Most importantly, the real policy initiative vanished when Ivan Lewis lost his post within the Department of Health. His strategy had been to use the development of personalisation as the means to radically reform the funding of adult social care. I resigned from my leadership of In Control in 2009, frustrated by the direction the whole process had taken.

'Zombie' personalisation

In practice, personalisation is now a mixture of the good, the bad and the ugly. Central government has a bad track record in implementing positive change, and when government decided that national leadership was 'essential', it was probably inevitable that we would end up with the expensive mess that personalisation has become.

Yet we cannot leave matters there. In 2010, the new coalition government introduced the most sweeping cuts to public services since the creation of the welfare state. And these cuts were not evenly spread; in particular, they targeted English local government (60% of whose function is social care) and benefits, including many disability benefits (Duffy, 2013b). For the first time in living memory, government policy seems to target disabled people for reductions in income and support.

What is surprising is to see that none of this has halted the apparent commitment of government to personalisation (Duffy, 2012a). Rather, personalisation has become one of the means by which cuts have been introduced. The resource allocation systems that were designed to empower people, it turns out, can equally be used to cut budgets. Costs are further cut by encouraging people to take their budgets as direct payments, sometimes without adequate support. And local authorities, in the name of efficiency and increased budgetary control, interfere in people's planning and decision making, drawing power back to the system (Duffy, 2012b).

At its worst, personalisation has become 'zombie' personalisation. The language and structures of self-directed support are used, but the underlying spirit is hostile to citizenship and hostile to community. Many of the institutions that proclaim the virtues of personalisation have found themselves so reliant on government funding that they cannot stand up for people or challenge what is going on.

I know that many individuals and families have benefited from personalisation, but many are also suffering because of personalisation – or at least because of what is now done in its name. It is now difficult to make any simple evaluation of personalisation simply because it is near impossible to distinguish the impact of personalisation from the impact of government cuts. If personalisation is now consistent with reducing the legal and economic rights of disabled people, clearly personalisation is just another tool of a neoliberal agenda to reduce the securities offered by the welfare state (Duffy, 2012d).

Lessons

Although this may seem to be a dispiriting story of unfulfilled promises, greed and confusion, there are some positive lessons that may be worth building on. For myself, these lessons are also an admission of failure (Duffy, 2012c). The In Control project promised so much and, for a short period, seemed to have achieved much; it is hard to accept that one's best efforts were wasted or misused. It is even harder to accept that you played a part in this yourself. But it is important to be as honest as possible about this and to try to avoid making similar mistakes in the future.

Citizenship is not a gift

The goal of personalisation was the advancement of citizenship. However, the means by which this goal was achieved was by the redesign of professional systems of control. In a sense, personalisation tried to change the Professional Gift Model into a Citizenship Model by stealth – by changing processes to encourage people to treat each other more like fellow citizens.

But today, as I look back on this effort, I wonder whether citizenship can ever really be achieved by stealth – simply by redesigning systems and processes. Indeed, historically, the battles for citizenship (from ancient Athens to women's suffrage, from a free India to black civil rights) have always been waged by citizens themselves – in their own name.

This truth appears all the more starkly in the light of the severe cuts that now target disabled people. And it is not just personalisation that has suffered this unexpected reverse. Many other important developments within government, such as the creation of the Office for Disability Issues, look very different when we find that government itself seeks to undermine the rights of disabled people.

What is more, many of the organisations that one would have expected to stand up for disabled people, such as charities, quangos and the media, have appeared spineless. Disabled people, families and their allies are going to need to develop much more robust political strategies in the future; they cannot rely on an assumption that the state will be benign or enlightened. It will be critical to establish constitutional protections, rooted in human rights (Chetty et al, 2012).

It is for this reason that developments such as the creation of the Campaign for a Fair Society or the Spartacus Network (an internet-based network of disabled researchers) are likely to become increasingly important (Campaign for a Fair Society, 2012). Political pressure and engagement with the real economic and legal rights of disabled people cannot be left to the system itself.

Tools are defined by their user

It is, of course, possible to argue that personalisation itself is fine – it is just being misused or misinterpreted by the system. But this is naive. Any tool or system will be defined by those who use it. Personalisation has allowed a whole range of such shifts in meaning:

- Resource allocation systems were designed to create robust and meaningful entitlements, but they are now used to rationalise unfair and unreasonable cuts.
- Person-centred planning systems were designed to help people to take control over their own decisions, but they are often used to justify more interference in people's lives.
- Individual budgets were designed to give people more control, without having to always directly manage the cash, but they are now used to pretend that people have control when they do not.
- Self-directed support was designed to create more flexibility, creativity and freedom, but too often it is used to tie people into complex contractual and regulatory systems.

This is not to say that all local authorities fail to implement self-directed support with integrity, but it does appear that the cuts have encouraged even more places to interpret self-directed support badly.

The greatest, and most worrying, ambiguity of self-directed support is that it may be well be used to worsen some of the other entitlements that people receive. Effectively, self-directed support created a system that sits half way between direct services (like acute surgery) and income adjustment (like benefits). Its purpose was to shift resources out of direct services and towards income (Duffy et al, 2010). Yet this direction of travel can be reversed. Many benefits are increasingly being made more conditional and bureaucratic, allowing sanctions or interference (Dwyer, 2010). It is quite possible that some will lobby for shifting benefits into the control of local authorities through the mechanism of self-directed support. This would be an even greater backward step.

Interestingly, none of this is necessary. The systems we use in our communities to ration resources, make decisions and keep each other safe can be developed in partnerships and can be freely shared and developed across our communities. Just as in the early days of In Control, before an excess of government funding washed away these structures, early pioneers in self-directed support freely shared their ideas and experiences. In fact, to develop together and share our tools may be an important dimension of a society that respects citizenship.

It is for this reason that networks of peer support – at every level – are important. When people work together, share ideas and support each other as fellow citizens, they can protect the integrity and value of what is important. Groups like Active Independence or the People Focused Group in Doncaster demonstrate a determination to remain in control of ideas and technologies and a refusal to let the system dictate their meaning (Duffy, 2013c).

Systems naturally resist reform

One of the most fascinating lessons of personalisation is that it has much to teach us about how change happens and how change is undermined (Duffy, 2013d). In fact, it is useful to realise that all systems resist change – this is natural and not from any malign intent – and that there are some reasonably predictable strategies that systems use to obstruct change:

- excluding innovation – the easiest way to avoid change is to deny the existence or relevance of any innovation. It is therefore very important to create changes that are not just theoretical but also become as real and as significant as possible;
- devaluing innovation – should an innovation take on a real and visible life, the next defensive strategy is to suggest there is no good evidence for it. So innovators must inevitably gather and share evidence in order to inspire others and overcome the system's natural scepticism;
- treating the innovation as an optional extra – if the innovation starts to feel inevitable, the system will try to add it on to its existing approaches as an appendix – something that is distinct from the rest of the system and does not appear to threaten it. This usually also has the impact of making the whole system more complicated and reducing the impact of the innovation. So the task of the innovator is to seek simplicity and efficiency – to make the innovation accessible and easy to use;

- obscuring the innovation – if the innovation becomes a required part of the system, the last defensive strategy is to so obscure the innovation so that it can be declared a success, without really changing anything. Yet for the innovator, the real challenge is to transform the system so the innovation really does disappear, by being integrated into a more effective system.

In the development of self-directed support, we were successful in the first two phases. However, I believe we largely failed to make the necessary breakthrough in the third and fourth phases. Today government and local authorities can declare personalisation a success, for they will be able to point to nearly one million people who have personal budgets. But in reality these budgets now form part of a system that does not empower people and where people's basic rights are hidden or denied.

This leaves us with some very fundamental challenges that go to the heart of the design and function of the welfare state. To make progress, we will need to combine a focus on innovation with a focus on the deeper structures that obstruct innovation (as shown in Figure 18.4). The tendency of the welfare system to stigmatise the disadvantaged, the centralisation of power by government and the growing levels of inequality in society all threaten positive change.

Figure 18.4: How innovations develop in public services

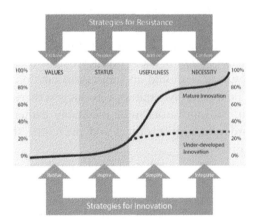

What next?

The welfare state is an essential part of a well-functioning and secure society. Yet, as we have seen, the system is under attack from those who deny its value while it struggles to meet the legitimate demands of ordinary people, especially the most disadvantaged. So, how do we reform something that we really need and yet is so difficult to improve? How do we transform the welfare state into something that is more secure, more innovative and more supportive of citizenship and community? I am going to end by offering three very practical thoughts, which could be relevant to any reader.

First, we must start with ourselves. If citizenship, community or social justice is important to you in your life or in your work, you must ask yourself how you are going to live by those values. This is possible in work, and it is possible within the welfare state, but it does require an honest evaluation of your own efforts and their meaning. Just following orders or doing what the system asks is not good enough. You must be a citizen, behave like a citizen – as if your actions matter and your community matters.

Second, focus on community. Even when systems are broken or badly designed, even when social injustice seems to be the order of the day, there is something you can do at the level of community. All the very best ideas and practices were dreamt up by men and women in communities trying to make things better. If you are inside the welfare system itself, ask yourself whether you know who is trying to do the right thing and what you can do to support them. If you feel alone, reach out – build community around you and your efforts.

Third, get political. There are currently millions of us who are badly affected by government policies and by the failures of the current system. Even when your paid role does not allow you to focus on these issues, you can act as a citizen in thinking, discussing, challenging, joining movements and ensuring that you and those you know are aware of your rights and aware of how to bring about political change.

Personalisation has arrived in the midst of the most difficult period in the history of the post-war welfare state. It is not the answer to our problems, but it does – for all its flaws – begin to ask some of the right questions. We do need systems that support citizenship – we cannot rely on paternalistic services to simply sweep us up and save the day. We do need community - welfare systems cannot replace family, friends or our fellow citizens. And we do need real rights, freedoms and duties and the opportunity to exercise them.

Personalisation has been an interesting phase in the history of the welfare state. It has shown the possibility of positive and radical change, and revealed its fragility. We must use this experience as we enter the next phase. After personalisation, there will be new efforts to reform the welfare system; it is to be hoped that these efforts will learn the lessons of personalisation.

NINETEEN

Conclusion:
glass half full or glass half empty?

Jon Glasby and Catherine Needham

Throughout history, most revolutions fail in the first instance. Some never really ignite and others end with a whimper in a short space of time. However, even revolutions that seem to be 'successful' at the time often fail to bring about anticipated results. Sometimes this is because previous elites are unwilling to give up power and find ways of going with the flow in the short term, but quietly re-emerge near the top of the new system. 'Turkeys do not vote for Christmas', as the popular saying goes, and it is rare to find a ruling group that voluntarily gives up power. On other occasions, the different groups demanding change can have much in common at a superficial level when united by a common enemy – but ultimately have different aims and objectives that become more apparent after the common enemy has been defeated. At the same time, many of the initial revolutionaries are charismatic or powerful personalities that others want to follow – but the same traits can make it easy for people to fall out after the event and for previously coherent movements to fragment amid significant jockeying and personality clashes.

This is probably an overly grandiose way to start the concluding chapter to this book – but many of the contributors to this edited collection do appear to suggest that the personalisation agenda has not led to the revolution (or at least to the subsequent long-term changes) that many people seem to have been hoping for. For Victoria Hart, personalisation has 'over-promised and has under-delivered', while Peter Beresford describes various potential 'traps'. For Simon Duffy, a key figure in the development of self-directed support, we have ended up with 'a mixture of the good, the bad and the ugly' at best – or '"zombie" personalisation' at worst. Moreover, some of the changes that have taken place under the banner of 'personalisation' might not only fail to deliver the positive changes anticipated, but could also actually make things worse. Thus, Helga Pile warns of the negative impact that there could be for staff and service users, Lucy Series describes a worrying lack of transparency and a series of legal tensions around resource allocation and Colin Slasberg debates a potential threat to the universalism of the NHS. Melanie Henwood identifies the difficulties that self-funders face, highlighting the point that people who already manage their own care arrangements do not necessarily receive high-quality services.

And yet, there is a danger of being overly negative. For all the barriers and problems identified in the different chapters in this collection, there are also many positives. Christine Bond talks passionately about the difference direct payments and personal budgets have made to her life, Colin Royle shows how personal health budgets restored the life of his family following his dad's dementia and Victoria Hart stresses how inspired many frontline workers are by the desire to support people using services to exercise much greater choice and control. Julien Forder and Karen Jones demonstrate how personal health budgets can improve outcomes, and Vidhya Alakeson only explores possible barriers because the potential of personal health budgets to make a positive difference seems to her so strong. Wendy Mitchell, Jenni Brooks and Caroline Glendinning show how personal budgets can have a positive effect for carers. Where some authors are wary, it is sometimes because personal budgets seem to have advantages for some groups, and the contributor is nervous that this may not be the case for everyone. Although this is an important issue, it is hardly a vote of no confidence in the concept of personalisation itself – more a plea that it should be designed and implemented in such a way that everyone can benefit. Despite identifying potential 'traps', Peter Beresford also explores lots of ways round them, and the Standards We Expect project is a wonderful example of the many changes needed to deliver more genuinely person-centred support.

Indeed, one of the interesting things for us has been the extent to which different contributors seem to agree on some of the underlying issues at stake. Although our introduction highlights the controversial and contested nature of the personalisation agenda, there has been less disagreement in practice than perhaps we were expecting. People may be writing from very different perspectives and taking different approaches to different aspects of the personalisation agenda, but they seem much more united than might first appear to be the case around a number of underlying principles. Throughout, many chapters are critical of a traditional system that they see as doing things to people (or even for them) rather than with them – and they argue for greater choice, control and independence. Often, these contributions seem to be influenced by an underlying citizenship or civil rights-based approach, with a fundamental belief that disabled and older people should have the same choices and the same degree of control over their lives as non-disabled people. Any fundamental disagreements that exist tend to centre on whether personalisation as currently conceived and implemented will help move us in the right direction and whether the potential risks are too great, and on the motives of key players and the likelihood of unintended consequences.

Against this background, why has the personalisation agenda been perceived by many here as failing to deliver and why are there differences in people's views as to what has/has not been achieved in practice? For us, a key part of the answer comes from Chapter Two, where we argued that part of personalisation's early appeal was its ability to unite people from across the political spectrum behind concepts of choice and independence. From the accounts in this edited collection, it is clear that 'personalisation' is a term that means different things to different people, but one that sounds inherently positive. It refers to something that is difficult to define, but that feels instinctively important – almost as if we don't quite know what personalisation means, but that if we didn't have the concept we would probably have to invent it. Elsewhere (see, for example, Glasby and Dickinson, 2014, p 3), we have argued that other buzzwords such as 'partnership', 'involvement' and 'community' play a similar function – conveying something positive and important in a way that few can argue against, but containing enough ambiguity to engage a range of different stakeholders in different ways.

In many ways, this can be seen as a key strength, leading to a broad appeal and significant momentum for change. However, once a new way of working is introduced, such ambiguity can prove frustrating as previous allies realise they may have been trying to achieve different things to each other and that they probably have less in common than they initially thought. Although it is a massive over-simplification, both direct payments and personal budgets were invented and promoted by people and organisations fundamentally committed to equal citizenship, to a rights-based agenda and to more fundamental social and political change. Yet the same concepts and policy mechanisms could also appeal to a neoliberal agenda that promotes individual rather than collective responsibility, a rolling back of the boundaries of the welfare state and a greater reliance on consumerism and market power. As Spandler (2004, p 202) observes:

> ... it seems clear that neither a simplistic pursuit of [direct payments] as empowerment, nor a kneejerk reaction against them as mere cost-cutting consumerism is an adequate response. [Direct payments] are not clearly a 'consumerist'

or a 'democratic' approach to social policy…, but actually an example of the convergence of the two, a convergence that yields both problems and possibilities.

Similarly, Sapey and Pearson (2004, p 65) suggest:

> Direct payments do make use of free market principles and there can be a contradiction between the individualism of this approach and the need for collectivity in the responsibility for welfare…. Direct payments need to be seen as an integral part of a collective approach to the provision of support. Implementing direct payment schemes provides a possibility of promoting independent living and access to mainstream economic and social life, but also could be a threat to collective responsibility for welfare and the notion of caring communities if it is interpreted within an individualist framework. The challenge is to do the first and not the second.

When we read the chapters in this book, many contributors seem disappointed that the current personalisation agenda seems to have lost touch with its initial roots and values, almost as if it has been hijacked by other stakeholders for purposes other than that for which it was intended. Going back to the opening to this chapter, this is not uncommon when revolutions take place; while many of the initial campaigners for a better world undoubtedly have pure motives, it is all too common for these initial movements to fragment and/or for their ideals to be co-opted by the current system and subtly diverted, diluted and undermined. For us, this is why Simon Duffy's notion of '"zombie" personalisation' is such an apt – if challenging – phrase. Perhaps unwittingly, we have seen something of a revolution in adult social care, only to find the old system reinvent itself under the guise of the new language and, in an era of austerity, leaving us with a shadow, a pale imitation or possibly even a parody of what personalisation could be. Whether you believe that personalisation is a 'Trojan horse' for neoliberalism or that a well-meaning policy has been 'derailed' (see p 21 of this book), the fact remains that there seem to be major problems and concerns with the current state of affairs.

At first glance, it is hard to imagine how the previous system could have reinvented itself, given the passionate commitment of so many people (including the authors in this book) to reforming and improving services. To a certain extent, this might be a case of unintended consequences, with widespread change difficult to achieve in complex bureaucracies where new approaches are often layered on existing systems, logics, targets and incentives. Simon Duffy also deals with this head-on with his discussion of ways in which change can be excluded, devalued, added on to existing systems and/or obscured so that very little changes in practice. For him, this is entirely natural and presumably a form of self-protection – but there is an inherent tendency for all systems to resist change. In recognition of this, he argues that nothing less than a new constitutional settlement, underpinned by a theory of citizenship and human rights, will be sufficient to bring about more fundamental reform. A similar point is made by Peter Beresford and others around the need to tackle the underlying funding settlement and overcome a 'deficit' model of social care if more widespread reform is to be achieved. It is often said that the particular systems are 'fundamentally broken' (see, for example, Glasby et al, 2013). Yet an alternative view would argue that all systems are perfectly designed to achieve the results they produce, and that more widespread change will need a genuine and society-wide commitment to producing something different and better for people using social care services.

Going forward, the different contributors to this book suggest a number of positive avenues (or ways of avoiding the 'traps' identified by Peter Beresford):

- First and foremost, several chapters identify potential barriers still to be tackled – but also stress how far the social care system has come over time. Rather than seeing personalisation as a one-off 'revolution', a number of contributors place more recent debates in a historical and/or a broader context, seeing personalisation as more of an evolutionary process and recognising the many changes which have slowly been taking place since the Seebohm report of 1968. It is partly this sense of personalisation as a journey rather than as an event that is behind the subtitle to this chapter. While recent changes are contentious, perhaps it depends on the timescales you adopt as to whether you take a 'glass half full' or a 'glass half empty' stance.
- Next is a recognition that choice and control are only meaningful when they go hand in hand with support. In a number of chapters, it is access to support that seems to have been crucial in making either direct payments or personal budgets a positive experience, whether this is Christine Bond's emphasis on the importance of peer support, Liz Lloyd's acknowledgement of the role of supportive family members and attentive professionals in enabling some older people to exercise greater choice or the focus of Wendy Mitchell

and colleagues on the crucial role played by carers. Towards the end of the book, Simon Duffy again stresses the importance of peer support at all levels of the system, while Peter Beresford's account and the Standards We Expect project are good illustrations of the way in which the collective voice of disabled people and their organisations has been such a powerful force for change. Equally, Melanie Henwood talks about what can happen when people funding their own care do not have sufficient access to meaningful advice and information.

• Perhaps even more important than support per se is the role of meaningful and trusting relationships. Although personalisation has prompted some to fear an excessive focus on individualism, the majority of chapters in this book focus in different ways on the importance of supportive relationships – whether with a peer, a family member, a service provider or a social worker. This ranges from Colin Royle's role in providing support to his father to Sian Lockwood's emphasis on the ingenuity and creativity of micro-enterprises and local communities. Simon Duffy stresses the importance of community, of basic social interaction and of acknowledging the unique skills and gifts that each person brings. Helga Pile also highlights the common cause that could be reasserted between the 'user' and the social care workforce, while Victoria Hart shows how passionate many social workers feel about seeing people thrive and be the best they can be. While personalisation could be about individual rather than collective responsibility, the chapters of this book paint a different picture, with a very real sense that 'we are all in it together'.

Above all, different commentators keep coming back to understanding and being clear about our own values and motives. If the aim for many contributors is greater social justice, a deeper sense of community and a more fundamental commitment to civil rights, direct payments, personal budgets and other ways of working as well are simply a means to an end. They may be potentially powerful approaches in their own right, but at the end of the day they are simply mechanisms. In a target-driven culture, there is a real risk that adult social care and other public services hit the target and miss the point – that they deliver the '"zombie" personalisation' described by Simon Duffy but that they ultimately fail to do anything meaningful to improve outcomes for people using services or to enhance independent living. For all their disagreements and differences in emphasis and interpretation, many of the contributors to this book seem united in calling for a more genuine and longer-lasting revolution in which direct payments and personal budgets are potentially only a small part of a broader change. In doing so, they are aware of how unconducive the current policy and financial context is to such a scenario – but they seem fundamentally committed to continuing to campaign for a better society and a better life together. Going back to our subtitle for this chapter, an optimist might look at things and say that the glass is half full. A pessimist might look at the same state of affairs and say that the glass is half empty. However, a key risk is that the Chancellor of the Exchequer and/or the local Director of Resources looks at the same situation and concludes that the glass is twice as big as it needs to be.

References

ACAS (2013) 'Disabled and elderly people and their personal assistants: the challenges of a unique employment relationship', ACAS, April 2013 www.acas.org.uk/media/pdf/j/l/Disabled-and-elderly-people-and-their-personal-assistants.pdf

ADASS (Association of Directors of Adult Social Services) (2010) *Common resource allocation framework*, London: ADASS.

ADASS (2013a) 'Social care funding: a bleak outlook is getting bleaker', Press Release, 8 May, www.adass.org.uk/Content/Article.aspx?id=1034

ADASS (2013b) 'ADASS survey shows personalised social services being offered to more and more users', Press Release, 10 September, www.adass.org.uk/index.php?option=com_content&view=article&id=931&Itemid=489

ADASS and RCPysch (Royal College of Psychiatrists) (2013) 'The integration of personal budgets in social care and personal health budgets in the NHS: Joint position statement', www.rcpsych.ac.uk/pdf/PS01_2013.pdf.

ADASS, Skills for Care and Centre for Workforce Intelligence (2013) 'Summary report of the workshop on direct payments and personal assistants: managing the emerging issues', www.skillsforcare.org.uk/nmsruntime/saveasdialog.aspx?lID=15569&sID=2681

Age UK (2011) *Care in crisis: Causes and solutions*, London: Age UK.

Alakeson, V. (2010) *Quality, innovation, productivity and prevention (QIPP) and personal health budgets*, Wythall: In Control Partnerships.

Alakeson, V. (2014) *Delivering personal health budgets: A guide to policy and practice*, Bristol: Policy Press.

Alakeson, V. and Duffy, S. (2011) *Health efficiencies: The possible impact of personalisation in healthcare*, Sheffield: The Centre for Welfare Reform.

Alakeson, V. and Perkins, R. (2012) *Recovery, personalisation and personal budgets*, London: Centre for Mental Health, www.mentalhealthuk.co.uk/pdf/CFMH%20Recovery%20Personalisation%20and%20PBH%20SEp%202012.pdf

Alakeson, V., Miller, C. and Bunin, A. (2013) *Coproduction of health and wellbeing outcomes: The new paradigm for effective health and social care*, London: Office for Public Management.

Alzheimer's Society (2011a) *Getting personal: Making personal budgets work for people with dementia*, London: Alzheimer's Society.

Alzheimer's Society (2011b) *Short changed: Protecting people with dementia from financial abuse*, London: Alzheimer's Society.

Arksey, H. and Glendinning, C. (2007) 'Choice in the context of informal care-giving', *Health and Social Care in the Community*, vol 15, no 2, pp 165-75.

Audit Commission (2010) *Financial management of personal budgets: Challenges and opportunities for local councils*, London: Audit Commission.

Audit Commission (2012a) *Reducing the cost of assessments and reviews: An adult social care briefing for councils*, London: Audit Commission.

Audit Commission (2012b) *Making personal health budgets sustainable: Practical suggestions on how to manage financial risk*, London: Audit Commission, www.bit.ly/1mdJg6G

Ball, S.J. (1997) 'Policy sociology and critical social research: a personal view of recent education policy and education policy research', *British Educational Research Journal*, vol 23, no 3, pp 257-74.

Barnes, M. (2011) 'Abandoning care? A critical perspective on personalisation from an ethic of care', *Ethics and Social Welfare*, vol 5, no 1, pp 153-67.

Barnes, M. (2012) *Care in everyday life: An ethic of care in practice*, Bristol: Policy Press.

Bartlett, J. (2009) *Getting more for less: Efficiency in the public sector*, London: Demos.

Baxter, K., Rabiee, P. and Glendinning, C. (2013) 'Managed personal budgets for older people: what are English local authorities doing to facilitate personalized and flexible care?', *Public Money & Management*, vol 33, no 6, pp 399-406.

BBC (2013) 'Jeremy Hunt highlights plight of "chronically lonely"', 18 October, www.bbc.co.uk/news/uk-politics-24572231

Bennett, S. (2012) *Personal health budgets guide: Implications for NHS-funded providers*, London: Department of Health.

Beresford, P. (2007) *The changing roles and tasks of social work from service users' perspectives: A literature informed discussion paper*, London: General Social Care Council.

Beresford, P. (2009) *Compass think piece 47: Whose personalisation?*, London: Compass.

Beresford, P. (2010) *A straight talking introduction to being a mental health service user*, Ross-on-Wye: PCCS Books.

Beresford, P. (2011a) 'Question marks surround Dilnot Commission proposals', *Community Care, The big picture*, 7 July, p 5.

Beresford, P. (2011b) 'Does the Dilnot Report go far enough?', *Society Guardian*, 4 July.

Beresford, P. (2012) 'Are personal budgets necessarily empowering for service users? If not, what's it all about?', *Research, Policy and Planning*, vol 29, no 1, pp 37-43.

Beresford, P. and Andrews, A. (2012) *Caring for our future: What service users say*, Programme Paper, York: Joseph Rowntree Foundation, www.jrf.org.uk/publications/caring-our-future-what-service-users-say

Beresford, P., Fleming, J., Glynn, M., Bewley, C., Croft, S., Branfield, F. and Postle, K. (2011) *Supporting people: Towards a person-centred approach*, Bristol: Policy Press.

BMA (British Medical Association) (2012) 'Government set to push ahead with personal health budgets', 2 November, http://bma.org.uk/news-views-analysis/news/2012/november/government-set-to-push-ahead-with-personal-health-budgets

Bottery, S. and Holloway, J. (2013) *Advice and information needs in adult social care*, Report for the Think Local, Act Personal partnership, London: Independent Age.

Boxall, K. Dowson, S. and Beresford, P. (2009) 'Selling individual budgets, choice and control: local and global influences on UK social care policy for people with learning difficulties', *Policy & Politics*, vol 37, no 4, pp 499-515.

Brissenden, S. (1986) 'Independent living and the medical model of disability', *Disability, Handicap and Society*, vol 1, no 2, pp 173-8.

Brooks, J., Mitchell, W. and Glendinning, C. (forthcoming) 'Personalisation, personal budgets and family carers: whose assessment? Whose budget?', *Health and Social Care in the Community*.

Burns, D., Hyde, P. and Killett, A. (2013) 'Wicked problems or wicked people? Reconceptualising institutional abuse', *Sociology of Health and Illness*, vol 35, no 4, pp 514-28.

Burton, M. (2013) 'Labour mulling social care tax, Burnham tells SOLACE', *Municipal Journal, The*, http://themj.co.uk/article/?id=195031&typeid=1.

Cameron, D. (2009) 'David Cameron: The Big Society', www.respublica.org.uk/item/ResPublica-mentioned-in-Camerons-speech-ggtc

Campaign for a Fair Society (2012) *Manifesto for a fair society 2012*, Sheffield: The Centre for Welfare Reform.

Carers UK (2008) *Choice or chore? Carers' experiences of direct payments*, London: Carers UK.

Carers UK (2010) *The coalition programme for government: What it means for carers*, London: Carers UK.

Carr, S. (2010) *Enabling risk, ensuring safety: Self-directed support and personal budgets*, London: Social Care Institute for Excellence.

Carr, S. (2012) 'Personalisation and marketisation: Policy construction and practice implementation – implications for third sector provision of adult social care and support in England', Paper presented at the International Society for Third Sector Research 10th International Conference, Siena, Italy, 10–13 July.

Carr, S. (2013) *Improving personal budgets for older people*, SCIE Adult Report 63, London: Social Care Institute of Excellence.

Carr-West, J. and Thraves, L. (2011) *Independent ageing: Council support for care self-funding*, London: Local Government Information Unit.

Charlesworth, A. and Thorlby, R. (2012) *Reforming social care: Options for funding*, London: Nuffield Foundation.

Chetty, K., Dalrymple, J. and Simmons, H. (2012) *Personalisation and human rights*, Sheffield: The Centre for Welfare Reform.

Clark, H., Dyer, S. and Horwood, J. (1998) *That bit of help: The high value of low level preventative services for older people*, Bristol: Policy Press.

Clarke, J., Newman, J., Smith, N., Vidler, E. and Westmarland, L. (2007) *Creating citizen-consumers: Changing publics and changing public services*, London: Sage Publications.

Clements, L. (2008) 'Individual budgets and irrational exuberance', *Community Care Law Reports*, vol 11, pp 413–30.

Clements, L., Bangs, J. and Holzhausen, E. (2009) 'Individual budgets and carers', www.lukeclements.co.uk/resources-index/files/PDF%20 05.pdf

Colebatch, H.K. (2005) 'Policy analysis, policy practice and political science', *Australian Journal of Public Administration*, vol 64, no 3, pp 14–23.

Collins, P. (2012) 'Saving Mrs Smith', *Prospect*, 14 November.

Community Care (2010) *The state of personalisation*, London: Community Care and UNISON.

Community Care (2011) *The state of personalisation*, London: Community Care and UNISON.

Community Care (2012) *The state of personalisation*, London: Community Care, UNISON and The College of Social Work.

Community Care (2013) *The state of personalisation*, London: Community Care.

Coulter, A. and Collins, A. (2011) *Making shared decision-making a reality: No decision about me, without me*, London: The King's Fund.

CSCI (Commission for Social Care Inspection) (2004) *Direct payments, what are the barriers?*, London: CSCI.

CSCI (2008a) *Cutting the cake fairly*, London: CSCI.

CSCI (2008b) *The state of social care in England 2006-07*, London: CSCI.

CSCI (2009) *The state of social care in England 2007-08*, London: CSCI.

Cutler, T., Waine, B. and Brehony, K. (2007) 'A new epoch of individualization? Problems with the "personalisation" of public sector services', *Public Administration*, vol 85, no 3, pp 847-55.

Darzi, A. (2007) *Our NHS, our future, NHS next stage review: Interim report*, London: Department of Health.

Darzi, A. (2008) *High quality care for all, NHS next stage review: Final report*, London: Department of Health.

Davidson, J., Baxter, K., Glendinning, C., Jones, K., Forder, J., Caiels, J., Welch, E., Windle, K. Dolan, P. and King, D. (2012) *Personal health budgets: Experiences and outcomes for budget holders at nine months. Fifth Interim Report*, London, Department of Health, http://php.york.ac.uk/inst/spru/pubs/2222/

Davison, S. and Rutherford, J. (2012) (eds) *Welfare Reform: The dread of things to come*, London, Lawrence Wishart.

Deeming, C. (2009) 'Active ageing in practice: a case study in East London, UK', *Policy &Politics*, vol 37, pp 93-111.

DH (Department of Health) (1998a) *Modernising social services promoting independence, improving protection, raising standards*, London: DH.

DH (1998b) *Community Care (Residential Accommodation) Act 1998*, LAC (98), London: DH.

DH (2002) *Fair access to care services: Guidance on eligibility criteria for adult social care*, LAC (13), London: DH.

DH (2005) *Independence, well-being and choice: Our vision for the future of social care for adults in England*, London: DH.

DH (2006) *Our health, our care, our say: A new direction for community services*, London: DH.

DH (2007) *Putting People First: A shared vision and commitment to the transformation of adult social care*, London: DH.

DH (2008) *Transforming social care*, LAC (1), London: DH.

DH (2009a) *Safeguarding adults: Report on the consultation on the review of 'No secrets'*, London: DH, http://webarchive.nationalarchives.gov.uk/+/www.dh.gov.uk/en/Consultations/Responsestoconsultations/DH_102764

DH (2009b) *The Community Care, Services for Carers and Children's Services (Direct Payments) (England) Regulations 2009*, London: DH.

DH (2009c) *Personal health budgets: First steps*, London, DH.

DH (2010a) *A vision for adult social care: Capable communities and active citizens*, London: DH.

DH (2010b) *Fairer contributions guidance: Calculating an individual's contribution to their personal budget*, London: DH.

DH (2010c) *Prioritising need in the context of Putting People First: A whole system approach to eligibility for social care: Guidance on eligibility criteria for adult social care, England 2010*, London: DH.

DH (2010d) *Practical approaches to safeguarding and personalisation*, London: DH, www.dh.gov.uk/prod_consum_dh/groups/dh_digitalassets/@dh/@en/@ps/documents/digitalasset/dh_121671.pdf.

DH (2010e) *Carers and personalisation: Improving outcomes*, London: DH.

DH (2010f) 'Mitchell's story', www.personalhealthbudgets.england.nhs.uk/Topics/latest/Resource/index.cfm?cid=7942.

DH (2010g) *Transparency in outcomes: A framework for adult social care*, London: DH.

DH (2012a) 'Personal health budgets to be rolled out', www.dh.gov.uk/health/2012/11/phb/

DH (2012b) *The adult social care outcomes framework 2013/14*, London: DH.

DH (2012c) *Caring for our future: Reforming care and support*, Cm 8378, London: The Stationery Office.

DH (2012d) *Long term conditions compendium of information* (3rd edn), London: DH.

DH (2012e) *Personal health budgets update*, London: DH.

DH (2012f) 'Government response to personal health budgets evaluation', www.personalhealthbudgets.england.nhs.uk/News/item/?cid=8606.

DH (2012g) *Understanding personal health budgets*, London: DH.

DH (2012h) *Transforming care: A national response to Winterbourne View Hospital. A Department of Health review: Final report*, London: DH.

DH (2013a) *The Care Bill explained: Including a response to consultation and pre-legislative scrutiny on the Draft Care and Support Bill*, London: The Stationery Office.

DH (2013b) *Policy statement on care and support funding reform and legislative requirements*, London: DH.

DH (2013c) *Draft national minimum eligibility threshold for adult care and support. A discussion document*, London: DH.

DH (2014) *Draft guidance on personal budgets*, London: DH.

DH/DCSF (2009) *Guidance on direct payment: For community care, services for carers and children's services*, London: DH, www.dh.gov.uk/prod_consum_dh/groups/dh_digitalassets/documents/digitalasset/dh_104895.pdf

Dilnot Commission (2011) *Fairer care funding: The report of the Commission on Funding of Care and Support*, London: Dilnot Commission.

Dixon, J., Manthorpe, J., Biggs, S., Tennant, R. and Mowlam, A. (2010) 'Defining elder abuse: reflections on the United Kingdom Study of the Abuse and Neglect of Older People', *Ageing and Society*, vol 30, no 3, pp 403-20.

Dixon, J., McNaughton-Nichols, C., D'Ardenne, J., Doyle, M. and Manthorpe, J. (2013) 'User involvement in designing a survey of people directly employing care and support workers', *Evidence and Policy*, vol 9, no 2, pp 267-78.

Donovan, T. (2012) 'Personal budgets increasingly bureaucratic, say professionals', *Community Care*, 4 July.

Duffy, S. (1992) 'Mutual accord', *Health Service Journal*, 102:5298.

Duffy, S. (1996) *Unlocking the imagination*, London: Choice Press.

Duffy, S. (2004) 'In control', *Journal of Integrated Care*, vol 12, no 6, pp 7-13.

Duffy, S. (2005a) 'Individual budgets: transforming the allocation of resources for care', *Journal of Integrated Care*, vol 13, no 1, pp 8-16.

Duffy, S. (2005b) *Individual budgets*, London: In Control Publications.

Duffy, S. (2006) *Keys to citizenship: A guide to getting good support for people with learning disabilities* (2nd edn), Sheffield: The Centre for Welfare Reform.

Duffy, S. (2010) 'The citizenship theory of social justice: exploring the meaning of personalisation for social workers', *Journal of Social Work Practice*, vol 24, no 3, pp 253-67.

Duffy, S. (2011a) *A fair income tax-benefit reform in an era of personalisation*, Birmingham: Health Services Management Centre, Centre for Welfare Reform.

Duffy, S. (2011b) 'Personalisation in social care - what does it really mean?', *Social Care and Neurodisability*, vol 2 no 4 pp 186-94.

Duffy, S. (2012a) 'The limits of personalisation', *Tizard Learning Disability Review*, vol 17, no 3, pp 110-23.

Duffy, S. (2012b) 'Personalisation or entitlements', *Community Living*, vol 25 no 4, www.centreforwelfarereform.org/library/by-date/personalisation-or-entitlements.html.

Duffy, S. (2012c) 'An apology', www.centreforwelfarereform.org/library/by-az/an-apology.html.

Duffy, S. (2012d) 'Is personalisation dead?', www.centreforwelfarereform.org/library/by-date/is-personalisation-dead.html.

Duffy, S. (2013a) *The unmaking of Man: Disability and the Holocaust*, Sheffield: The Centre for Welfare Reform.

Duffy, S. (2013b) *A fair society? How the cuts target disabled people*, Sheffield: The Centre for Welfare Reform.

Duffy, S. (2013c) *Whose community is it anyway? Rethinking the commissioning of user-led organisations and centres for independent living*, Sheffield: The Centre for Welfare Reform.

Duffy, S. (2013d) 'Forty years of innovation in community responses to the needs of people with learning difficulties', in C. Davies, J. Walmsley, M. Hales and R. Flux (eds) *Better health in harder times*, Bristol: Policy Press, pp 149-152.

Duffy, S. and Fulton, K. (2009) *Should we ban brokerage?*, Sheffield: The Centre for Welfare Reform.

Duffy, S. and Fulton, K. (2010) *Architecture for personalisation*, Sheffield: The Centre for Welfare Reform.

Duffy, S. and Sanderson, H. (2005) 'Relationships between care management and person centred planning', in P. Cambridge and S. Carnaby (eds) *Person centred planning and care management with people with learning disabilities*, London: Jessica Kingsley Publishers, pp 34-50.

Duffy, S., Waters, J. and Glasby, J. (2010) 'Personalisation and adult social care: future options for the reform of public services', *Policy and Politics*, vol 38, no 4, pp 493-508.

Duffy, S., Waters, J. and Glasby, J. (2010) *Personalisation and the social care revolution: Future options for the reform of public services*, Health Services Management Centre Policy Paper 3, Birmingham: University of Birmingham, Health Services Management Centre.

Dunn, M.C., Clare, I.C. and Holland, A. J. (2008) 'To empower or to protect? Constructing the "vulnerable adult" in English law and public policy', *Legal Studies*, 28, no 2, pp 234-53.

Dunning, J. (2011) 'Cuts are ravaging personalisation, say social workers', *Community Care*, 28 January, www.communitycare. co.uk/2011/01/28/cuts-are-ravaging-personalisation-say-social-workers/#.U8lL-vldUXw.

Dwyer, P. (2010) *Understanding social citizenship*, Bristol: Policy Press.

Ehlers, A., Naegele, G. and Reichert, M. (2011) *Volunteering by older people in the EU*, Dublin: European Foundation for the Improvement of Living and Working Conditions.

EHRC (Equality and Human Rights Commission) (2011) *Close to home: An inquiry into older people and human rights in home care*, London: EHRC.

Ellis, K. (2013) 'Professional discretion and adult social work: exploring its nature and scope on the frontline of personalisation', *British Journal of Social Work*, doi: 1-.1093/bjsw/bct076.

Epstein, R.M., Fiscella, K., Lesser, C.S. and Stange, K.C. (2010) 'Why the nation needs a policy push on patient-centered health care', *Health Affairs*, vol 29, no 8, pp 1489-95.

Evans, S.E. (2004) *Forgotten crimes: The Holocaust and people with disabilities*, Chicago, IL: Ivan R Dee.

Falkingham, J., Evadrou, M., McGowan, T. et al (2010) *Demographic issues, projections and trends: Older people with high support needs in the UK*, York: Joseph Rowntree Foundation.

Fawcett, B. (2012) 'Well-being and older people: the place of day clubs in reconceptualising participation and challenging deficit', *British Journal of Social Work*, doi: 10.1093/bjsw/bcs145.

Fenton, W. (2011) *The size and structure of the adult social care sector and workforce in England*, Leeds: Skills for Care.

Ferguson, I. (2007) 'Increasing user choice or privatizing risk: the antimonies of personalization', *British Journal of Social Work*, vol 37, pp 387-403.

Ferguson, I. (2008) *Reclaiming Social Work: Challenging Neo-Liberalism and Promoting Social Justice*, London: Sage.

Ferguson, I. (2012) 'Personalisation, social justice and social work: a reply to Simon Duffy', *Journal of Social Work Practice: Psychotherapeutic Approaches in Health, Welfare and the Community*, vol 26, no 1, pp 55-73.

Fine, M. and Glendinning, C. (2005) 'Dependence, independence or interdependence? Revisiting the concepts of "care" and "dependency"', *Ageing and Society*, vol 25, no 4, pp 601-21.

Fischer, F. (2003) *Reframing public policy: Discursive politics and deliberative practices*, Oxford: Oxford University Press.

Fitzpatrick, J. (2010) *Personalised support: How to provide high quality support to people with complex and challenging needs. Learning from Partners for Inclusion*, Sheffield: Centre for Welfare Reform.

Flynn, M. (2005) *Developing the role of personal assistants*, Leeds: Skills for Care.

Forder, J., Jones K., Glendinning, C., Caiels, J., Welch, E., Baxter, K., Davidson, J., Windle, K., Irvine, A., King, D. and Dolan, P. (2012) *Evaluation of the Personal Health Budget Pilot Programme*, London: DH, http://php.york.ac.uk/inst/spru/pubs/2331/

Fox, A. (2011a) 'Myths, cynicism and personalisation', Blog post, 10 April, http://alexfoxblog.wordpress.com/2011/04/10/myth/

Fox, A. (2011b) 'Time to ditch the RAS', Blog post, 5 July, http://alexfoxblog.wordpress.com/2011/07/05/time-to-ditch-the-ras/

Francis, J., Fisher, M. and Rutter, D. (2011) *Reablement: A cost-effective route to better outcomes*, Research Briefing 36, London: Social Care Institute for Excellence.

Francis, R. (2013) *Report of the Mid Staffordshire NHS Foundation Trust Public Inquiry*, London: The Stationery Office.

Gadsby, E. (2013) *Personal health budgets: A review of the evidence*, Canterbury: Centre for Health Studies, University of Kent.

Gallie, W. B. (1955) 'Essentially contested concepts', in *Proceedings of the Aristotelian Society, Vol. 56*, London: Blackwell Publishing, pp 167-98.

Glasby, J. (2007) *Understanding health and social care*, Bristol: Policy Press.

Glasby, J. (2012a) 'The controversies of choice and control: why some people might be hostile to English social care reform', *British Journal of Social Work*, 1-15 (doi: 10.1093/bjsw/bcs125).

Glasby, J. (2012b) *Whose risk is it anyway? Risk and regulation in an era of personalisation*, York: Joseph Rowntree Foundation, www.jrf.org.uk/sites/files/jrf/personalisation-service-users-risk-full.pdf

Glasby, J., Alakeson, V. and Duffy, S. (2014) *Doctor knows best? The use of evidence in implementing self directed support in health care*, Birmingham: Health Services Management Centre.

Glasby, J. and Dickinson, H. (2014) *Partnership working in health and social care: What is integrated care and how can we deliver it?* (2nd edn), Bristol: Policy Press.

Glasby, J. and Littlechild, R. (2006) 'An overview of the implementation and development of direct payments', in J. Leece and J. Bornat (eds) *Developments in direct payments*, Bristol: Policy Press, pp 19-32.

Glasby, J. and Littlechild, R. (2009) *Direct payments and personal budgets: Putting personalisation into practice* (2nd edn), Bristol: Policy Press.

Glasby, J., Le Grand, J. and Duffy, S. (2009) 'A healthy choice? Direct payments and healthcare in the English NHS', *Policy & Politics*, vol 37, no 4, pp 481-97.

Glasby, J., Miller, R. and Lynch, J. (2013) *Turning the welfare state upside down? Developing a new adult social care offer*, Policy Paper 15, Birmingham: Health Services Management Centre, University of Birmingham, in association with Birmingham City Council.

Glendinning, C., Challis, D., Fernandez, J.-L., Jacobs, S., Jones, K., Knapp, M., Manthorpe, J., Moran, N., Netten, A., Stevens, M. and Wilberforce, M. (2008) *Evaluation of the individual budgets pilot programme*, York: Social Policy Research Unit, University of York.

Glendinning, C., Arksey, H., Jones, K., Moran, N., Netten, A. and Rabiee, P. (2009) *The individual budgets pilot projects: Impact and outcomes for carers*, York: Social Policy Research Unit, University of York.

Glendinning, C., Moran, N., Challis, D., Fernandez, J.-L., Jacobs, S., Jones, K., Knapp, M., Manthorpe, J., Netten, A., Stevens, M. and Wilberforce, M. (2011) 'Personalisation and partnership: competing objectives in English adult social care? The individual budget pilot projects and the NHS', *Social Policy and Society*, vol 10, no 2, pp 151-62.

Goldberg, D. (1992) *General Health Questionnaire*, Windsor: NFER Nelson.

Grootegoed, E., Knijn, T. and da Roit, B. (2010) 'Relatives as paid care-givers: how family carers experience payments for care', *Ageing and Society*, vol 30, no 3, pp 467–89.

Hajer, M. (1995) *The politics of environmental discourse: Ecological modernization and the policy process*, Oxford: Oxford University Press.

Hall, S. (2003) 'New Labour's double shuffle', *Soundings*, vol 24, pp 10–24.

Harding, T. and Beresford, P. (eds) (1996) *The Standards We Expect: What service users and carers want from social services workers*, London: National Institute for Social Work.

Hasler, F. (2013) *Trust is the key: Increasing the take up of direct payments*, London: TLAP

Hatton, C. (2013) 'Fight the power? Personalisation and power in England', In Control Blog, 14 October, www.in-control.org.uk/blog/fight-the-power-personalisation-and-power-in-england.aspx

Hatton, C. and Slasberg, C. (2011) 'Personalisation: are personal budgets improving outcomes?', *Community Care*, 30 September, www.communitycare.co.uk/articles/30/09/2011/117526/personalisation-are-personal-budgets-improving-outcomes.htm

Hatton, C. and Waters, J. (2011) *The National Personal Budget Survey, June 2011*, Think Local, Act Personal, London: In Control Publications.

Hatton, C. and Waters, J. (2013) *Second National Personal Budget Survey*, Think Local, Act Personal, London: In Control Publications.

Health Foundation (2010) *Personal health budgets: Research scan*, London: Health Foundation.

Henwood, M. (2011), 'Journeys without maps: The decisions and destinations of people who self-fund', in *People who pay for care: Quantitative and qualitative analysis of self-funders in the social care market*, London: Putting People First Consortium, pp 43–83, www.bit.ly/1r0Eubx

Henwood, M. and Hudson, B. (2007) *Here to stay? Self-directed support: Aspiration and implementation: A review for the Department of Health*, Towcester: Melanie Henwood Associates.

HM Government (2008) *Carers at the heart of 21st century families and communities*, London: HM Government.

HM Government (2010) *Recognised, valued and supported: Next steps for the Carers' Strategy*, London: The Stationery Office.

HM Government (2012) *Caring for Our Future: White Paper*, London. The Stationery Office.

House of Commons (2009) 'Memorandum by Diabetes UK: NHS next stage review, www.publications.parliament.uk/pa/cm200809/cmselect/cmhealth/53/53we16.htm.

House of Commons (2013) 'Written statements', 8 October, www.publications.parliament.uk/pa/cm201314/cmhansrd/cm131008/wmstext/131008m0001.htm#131008m0001.htm_spmin12.

House of Lords (2013a) 'Are we ready for ageing? Report of the Select Committee on Public Service and Demographic Change', www.publications.parliament.uk/pa/ld201213/ldselect/ldpublic/140/14003.htm

House of Lords (2013b) *Hansard*, 29 October, column 1468.

HSCIC (Health and Social Care Information Centre) (2012) *Personal social services: Expenditure and unit costs, England 2010-11, Final Release*, www.ic.nhs.uk

Hudson, B. and Henwood, M. (2008) *Prevention, personalisation and prioritisation in social care: Squaring the circle?*, London: Centre for Social Care Excellence.

Hudson, B. and Henwood, M. (2009) *A parallel universe? People who fund their own care and support: A review of the literature*, London: Putting People First Consortium.

Humphries, R., Forder, J. and Fernandez, J.-L. (2010) *Securing good care for more people: Options for reform*, London: The King's fund.

Hunter, S., Manthorpe, J., Ridley, J., Cornes, M. and Rosengard, A. (2012) 'When self-directed support meets adult support and protection: findings from the evaluation of the SDS test sites in Scotland', *Journal of Adult Protection*, vol 14, no 4, pp 206-15.

International Futures Forum (2011) *Transforming finance*, 19 February, www.internationalfuturesforum.com/s/195

IPC Institute of Public Care (2011) 'Estimating the numbers and distribution of self-funders of care in England', *People who pay for care: quantitative and qualitative analysis of self-funders in the social care market*, London, Putting People First Consortium.

Jackson, V. and Duffy, S (2009) 'Collaboration and innovation: Oldham and In Control' in *More than good ideas: The power of innovation in local government*, London, IDeA.

Jacobs, S., Abell, J., Stevens, M., Wilberforce, M., Challis, D., Manthorpe, J., Fernandez, J.,

Glendinning, C., Jones, K., Knapp, M., Moran, N. and Netten, M. (2011) 'The personalisation of care services and the early impact on staff activity patterns', *Journal of Social Work*, vol 13, no 2, pp 141-63.

Jerome, J. (2010) Speech at the In Control Big Event, Liverpool, 15 March, www.in-control.org.uk/bigevent2010audio.

Johnson, F. (2102) 'Problems with the term and concept of "abuse": critical reflections on the Scottish Adult Support and Protection Study', *British Journal of Social Work*, vol 42, no 5, pp 833-50.

Johnson, S. (2013) 'Patient feedback to drive change across the health service', Guardian Healthcare Professionals Network, www.theguardian.com/healthcare-network/2013/oct/31/nhs-patient-feedback-change.

Jones, K., Netten, A., Rabiee, P., Glendinning, C., Arksey, H. and Moran, N. (2012) 'Can individual budgets have an impact on carers and the caring role?', *Ageing and Society*, doi:10.1017/S0144686X12000748.

Kittay, E.F. (2002) 'When caring is just and justice is caring: caring and mental retardation', in E.F. Kittay and E.K. Feder (eds) *The subject of care: Feminist perspectives on dependency*, Lanham, MD: Rowman and Littlefield.

Klee, D. and Williams, C. (2013) *Making Safeguarding Personal*, London: Local Government Association.

Kröger, T. (2009) 'Care research and disability studies: nothing in common?', *Critical Social Policy*, vol 29, no 3, pp 398-420.

Lamb, N. (2013) 'Personal health budgets', www.publications.parliament.uk/pa/cm201314/cmhansrd/cm131008/wmstext/131008m0001.htm#131008m0001.htm_spmin12.

Law Commission (2008) *Adult social care: A scoping report*, London: Law Commission.

Law Commission (2011) *Adult social care*, HC 941, London: The Stationery Office.

Leadbeater, C. (2004) *Personalisation through participation: A new script for public services*, London: Demos.

Leadbeater, C., Bartlett, J. and Gallagher, N. (2008) *Making it personal*, London: Demos.

Lloyd, J. (2013) *A cap that fits: The 'capped cost plus' model*, London: Strategic Society Centre.

Lloyd, L. (2010) 'The individual in social care: the ethics of care and the "personalisation agenda" in services for older people in England', *Ethics and Social Welfare*, vol 4, no 2, pp 188-200.

Lloyd, L., Calnan, M., Cameron, A., Seymour, J. and Smith, R. (2012) 'Identity in the fourth age: perseverance, adaptation and maintaining dignity', *Ageing and Society*, vol 1, no 1, pp 1-19.

London Borough of Newham (2009) *LBN risk enablement panel*, London: London Borough of Newham, www.dhcarenetworks.org.uk/Personalisation/Topics/Browse/Risk/?parent=3151&child=5007

Lymbery, M. (2012) 'Social work and personalisation', *British Journal of Social Work*, vol 42, no 4, pp 783-92.

Manthorpe, J. and Moriarty, J. (2010) *Nothing ventured, nothing gained*, London: Department of Health, www.dh.gov.uk/prod_consum_dh/ groups/dh_digitalassets/@dh/@en/@ps/documents/digitalasset/ dh_121493.pdf

Manthorpe, J. and Samsi, K. (2013) '"Inherently risky?": Personal budgets for people with dementia and the risks of financial abuse: findings from an interview-based study with adult safeguarding coordinators', *British Journal of Social Work* , vol 43, no 5, pp 889-903.

Manthorpe, J., Stevens, M., Rapaport, J., Harris, J., Jacobs, S., Challis, D., Netten, A., Knapp, M., Wilberforce, M. and Glendinning C. (2009) 'Safeguarding and system change: early perceptions of the implications for adult protection services of the English individual budgets pilots – a qualitative study', *British Journal of Social Work*, vol 29, no 8, pp 1465-80.

Manthorpe, J., Rapaport, J., Challis, D., Jacobs, S., Netten, A., Jones, K., Knapp, M., Wilberforce, M. and Glendinning, C. (2011) 'Individual budgets and adult safeguarding: parallel or converging tracks? Further findings from the evaluation of the individual budget pilots', *Journal of Social Work*, vol 11, no 4, pp 422-38.

Manthorpe, J., Williams, C., Klee, D. and Cooper, A. (2014) 'Making Safeguarding Personal: developing responses and enhancing skills', *Journal of Adult Protection*, vol 16, no 2, pp 96-103.

Manthorpe, J., Samsi, K. and Chandaria, K. (in press) 'Risks of financial abuse of older people with dementia: findings from a survey of UK voluntary sector dementia community services staff', *Journal of Adult Protection*.

Mathers, N., Thomas, M. and Patel, V. (2012) *Personal health budgets: RCGP position statement*, London: Royal College of General Practitioners.

Means, R. (2012) 'A brave new world of personalized care? Historical perspectives on social care and older people in England', *Social Policy and Administration*, vol 46, no 3, pp 302-20.

Miller, C., Bunnin, A. and Rayner, V. (2013) *Older people who self fund their social care: A guide for health and wellbeing boards and commissioners*, London: OPM.

Mitchell, W. (2012) 'Making choices about medical interventions: the experiences of disabled young people with degenerative conditions', *Health Expectations*, doi:10.111/j.1369-7625.2011.00752.x.

Mitchell, W., Brooks, J. and Glendinning, C. (2014) 'Carers roles in personal budgets: tensions and dilemmas in frontline practice', *British Journal of Social Work*.

Moran, N., Glendinning, C., Stevens, M., Manthorpe, J., Jacobs, S., Wilberforce, M., Knapp, M., Challis, D., Fernández J.-L., Jones, K. and Netten, A. (2011) 'Joining up government by integrating funding streams? The experiences of the individual budget pilot projects for older and disabled people in England', *International Journal of Public Administration*, vol 34, no 4, pp 232-43.

Moran, N., Arksey, H., Glendinning, C., Jones, K., Netten, A. and Rabiee, P. (2012) 'Personalisation and carers: whose rights? Whose benefits?', *British Journal of Social Work*, vol 42, no 3, pp 461-79.

Morris, J. (1993) *Independent lives: Community care and disabled people*, Basingstoke: Macmillan.

Mount, B. (1987) *Person-centred planning*, New York, NY: Graphic Futures.

NAO (National Audit Office) (2011) *Oversight of user choice and provider competition in care markets: Report by the Comptroller and Auditor General, summary*, London: The Stationery Office.

NAO (2013) *Emergency admissions to hospital: Managing the demand*, London: The Stationery Office.

Needham, C. (2010a) *Commissioning for personalisation: From the fringes to the mainstream*, London: Public Management and Policy Association.

Needham, C (2010b) 'Personalisation: from storyline to practice', *Journal of Social Policy & Administration*, vol 45, no 1, pp54-68.

Needham, C (2011a) *Personalising public services: Understanding the personalisation narrative*, Bristol: Policy Press.

Needham, C. (2011b) 'Personalisation: from storyline to practice', *Journal of Social Policy and Administration*, vol 45, no 1, pp 54-68.

Needham, C. (2012) *What is happening to day centre services? Voices from frontline staff*, Birmingham: Health Services Management Centre, University of Birmingham and UNISON.

Needham, C. (2013) 'Personalisation: from day centres to community hubs?', *Critical Social Policy*, vol 34, no 1, pp 47-65.

Netten, A., Burge, P., Malley, J., Potoglou, D., Towers, A.-M., Brazier, J., Fynn, T., Forder, J. and Wall, B. (2012) 'Outcomes of social care for adults: developing a preference-weighted measure', *Health Technology Assessment*, no 16, pp 1-165.

Newbronner, L., Chamberlain, R., Bosanquet, K., Bartlett, C., Sass, B. and Glendinning, C. (2011) *Keeping personal budgets personal: Learning from the experiences of older people, people with mental health problems and their carers*, Adult Services Report 40, London: Social Care Institute for Excellence.

Newman, J., Glendinning, C. and Hughes, M. (2008) 'Beyond modernisation? Social care and the transformation of welfare governance', *Journal of Social Policy*, vol 37, no 4, pp 531–57.

NHS Choices (2013) 'Principles and values that guide the NHS', www.nhs.uk/NHSEngland/thenhs/about/Pages/nhscoreprinciples.aspx.

NHS England (2013) 'Personal health budgets', www.personalhealthbudgets.england.nhs.uk/About/faqs/.

NICE (National Institute for Health and Clinical Excellence) (2007) *Briefing paper for the methods working party on the cost effectiveness threshold*, London: NICE.

Nicholson, C., Meyer, J., Flatley, M., Homan, C. and Lowton, K. (2012) 'Living on the margin: understanding the experience of living and dying with frailty in old age', *Social Science and Medicine*, vol 75, pp 1426–32.

NMHDU (National Mental Health Development Unit) (2011) *Facing up to the challenge of personal health budgets: The view of frontline professionals*, London: NHS Confederation.

Nuffield Council on Bioethics (2009) 'Dementia: ethical issues', www.nuffieldbioethics.org/fileLibrary/pdf/Dementia_report_for_web.pdf

O'Brien, J. (1991) *More than just a new address*, Lithonia: GA Responsive Systems Associates.

O'Brien, J. and Blessing, C. (eds) (2011) *Citizenship and person-centred work*, Toronto: Inclusion Press.

O'Brien, J. and Duffy, S. (2009) 'Self-directed support as a framework for partnership working', in J. Glasby and H. Dickinson (eds) *International perspectives on health and social care*, Chichester: Blackwell Publishing.

O'Brien, J. and Lyle O'Brien, C. (1998) *A little book about person centered planning*, vol 1, Toronto: Inclusion Press.

ODI (Office for Disability Issues) (2008) *Independent living: A cross-government strategy about independent living for disabled people*, London: The Stationery Office

OECD (Organisation for Economic Co-operation and Development) (2005) *Long-term care for older people*, Paris: OECD Publishing.

Oliver, M. (1990) *The politics of disablement*, Basingstoke: Macmillan.

Oliver, M. (1996) *Understanding disability: From theory to practice*, Basingstoke: Macmillan.

ONS (Office for National Statistics) (2012) *Mortality in the United Kingdom, 2010*, London: Office for National Statistics, www.ons.gov.uk/ons/dcp171780_251270.pdf

Osborne, L. (2013) 'Pensioner forced to pay £3,500 in compensation to carer for constructive dismissal because her hours were cut when his wife died', *Daily Mail*, 23 October.

Pickard, L. (2004) *The effectiveness and cost-effectiveness of support and services to informal carers of older people*, London: Audit Commission.

Pile, H. (2013) *All in the name of personalisation*, in P. Beresford (ed) *Personalisation*, Bristol: Policy Press, pp 65-69.

PMSU (Prime Minister's Strategy Unit)(2005) *Improving the life chances of disabled people*, London: Cabinet Office.

Podro, S. (2013) *Disabled and elderly people and their personal assistants: The challenges of a unique employment relationship*, ACAS.

Poll, C. and Duffy, S. (eds) (2008) *A report on In Control's second phase: Evaluation and learning 2005-2007*, London: In Control Publications.

Poll, C., Duffy, S., Hatton, C., Sanderson, H. and Routledge, M. (2006) *A report on In Control's first phase 2003-2005*, London: In Control Publications.

Pollitt, C. (2003) 'Joined-up government: a survey', *Political Studies Review*, vol 1, no 1, pp 34-49.

Princess Royal Trust for Carers and Crossroads Care (2010) *No breaks for carers: A report on primary care trusts and delivery of the national carers' strategy*, London: Princess Royal Trust for Carers and Crossroads Care.

Purdy, S. (2010) *Avoiding hospital admissions: What does the research evidence say?*, London: The Kings Fund.

Race, D. (2007) *Intellectual disability*, Maidenhead: Open University Press.

Raftery, J. (2009) 'NICE and the challenge of cancer drugs', *British Medical Journal*, 338:b67.

Rawls, J. (1971) *A theory of justice*, Oxford: Oxford University Press.

Repper, J. and Carter, T. (2010) 'A review of the literature on peer support in mental health services', *Journal of Mental Health*, vol 20, no 4, pp 392-411.

Repper, J. and Perkins, R. (2003) *Social inclusion and recovery: A model for mental health practice*, London: Baillière Tindall.

Roberts, A., Marshall, L. and Charlesworth, A. (2012) *A decade of austerity?*, London: Nuffield Trust.

Roulstone, A. and Prideaux, S. (2012) *Understanding disability policy*, Bristol: Policy Press.

Routledge, M. (2010) Speech at the In Control Big Event, Liverpool, 15 March, www.in-control.org.uk/bigevent2010audio

Routledge, M. (2011) 'Let's not allow bureaucracy to derail personalisation', *Community Care*, 25 May.

Routledge, M. and Carr, S. (2013) *Improving personal budgets for older people: A review. Phase one report*, London: Think Local, Act Personal.

Samsi, K., Manthorpe, J. and Chandaria, K. (2014) 'Risks of financial abuse of older people with dementia: findings from a survey of UK voluntary sector dementia community services staff', *Journal of Adult Protection*, vol 16, no 3, pp 71–83.

Samuel, M. (2010) 'Personalisation losing favour among social workers', *Community Care*, 20 May.

Samuel, M. (2012) 'Lamb scraps 100% personal budgets target', *Community Care*, 26 October.

Samuel, M. (2013a) 'Most councils met 70 percent personal budgets target, say directors', *Community Care*, 9 September.

Samuel, M. (2013b) 'Red tape and lack of funding limit choice for people on council-managed personal budgets', *Community Care*, 8 October.

Sapey, B. and Pearson, C. (2004) 'Do disabled people need social workers?', *Social Work and Social Sciences Review*, vol 11, no 3, pp 52-70.

SCIE (Social Care Institute for Excellence in conjunction with Carers UK) (2009) *Personalisation briefing: Implications for carers*, London: SCIE.

Scourfield, P. (2005) 'Implementing the Community Care (Direct Payments) Act: will the supply of personal assistants meet the demand and at what price?', *Journal of Social Policy*, vol 34, no 3, pp 469-88.

Scourfield, P. (2007) 'Social care and the modern citizen: client, consumer, service user, manager and entrepreneur', *British Journal of Social Work*, vol 37, no 1, pp 107-22.

Secretary of State for Health (2013) *The Care Bill explained including a response to consultation and pre-legislative scrutiny on the draft Care and Support Bill*, London: HMSO.

Series, L. and Clements, L. (2013) 'Putting the cart before the horse: resource allocation systems and community care', *Journal of Social Welfare and Family Law*, vol 35, no 2, pp 207-26.

Shakespeare, T. (2000) 'The social relations of care', in G. Lewis, S. Gewirtz and J. Clarke (eds) *Rethinking social policy*, Thousand Oaks: CA: Sage Publications, pp 52-65.

Skills for Care (2013) *The size and structure of the adult social care sector and workforce in England*, Leeds: Skills for Care

Slasberg, C., Beresford, P. and Schofield, P. (2012a) 'How self directed support is failing to deliver personal budgets and personalisation', *Research, Policy and Planning*, vol 29, no 3, pp 161-77.

Slasberg, C., Beresford, P. and Schofield, P. (2012b) 'Can personal budgets really deliver better outcome for all at no cost? Reviewing the evidence, costs and quality', *Disability & Society*, vol 27, no 7, pp 1029-34.

Slasberg, C., Beresford, P. and Schofield, P. (2013) 'The increasing evidence of how self-directed support is failing to deliver personal budgets and personalisation', *Research, Policy and Planning*, vol 30, no 2, pp 91–106.

Slasberg, C., Watson, N., Beresford, P. and Schofield, P. (2014) 'Personalisation of health in the UK: have the wrong lessons been drawn from the personal health budget pilots?', *Journal of Health Services Research and Policy*, doi: 10.1177/1355819614527577.

Slay, J. (2010) Budge*ts and Beyond: Interim report. A review of the literature on personalisation and a framework for understanding co-production in the 'Budgets and Beyond' project*, Produced for the Social Care Institute for Excellence, London: New Economics Foundation.

Spandler, H. (2004) 'Friend or foe? Towards a critical reassessment of direct payments', *Critical Social Policy*, vol 24, no 2, pp 187–209.

Spicker, P. (2012) 'Personalisation falls short', *British Journal of Social Work*, pp 1–17, doi:10.1093/bjsw/bcs063.

Stansfield, J. (2013) 'Are social care personal budgets working?', *The Guardian*, www.guardian.co.uk/society/2013/feb/12/are-social-care-personal-budgets-working

Sullivan, H. (2011) '"Truth" junkies: using evaluation in UK public policy', *Policy & Politics*, vol 39 no 4, pp 499–512.

Teater, B. and Baldwin, M. (2012). 'Singing for successful ageing: the perceived benefits of participating in the Golden Oldies community-arts programme', *British Journal of Social Work*, pp 1–19, doi:10.1093/bjsw/bcs095.

Teather, S. (2012) 'Special educational needs reform: draft legislation published', www.education.gov.uk/childrenandyoungpeople/send/changingsen/b00213564/wms-sen-reform

TLAP (Think Local, Act Personal) (2011a) *Minimum process framework*, London: TLAP.

TLAP (2011b) *Think Local, Act Personal: A sector-wide commitment to moving forward with personalisation and community-based support*, London: TLAP.

TLAP (2011c) *Making it real: Marking progress towards personalised, community based support*, London: TLAP.

TLAP (2013a) *National Personal Budgets Survey 2013*, London: TLAP, www.thinklocalactpersonal.org.uk/_library/POETSummaryFinal.pdf

TLAP (2013b) *Principles for the provision of information and advice*, London: TLAP.

Towell, D. (ed) (1988) *An ordinary life in practice*, London: The King's Fund.

Tu, T., Lambert, C., Shah, J.N., Westwood, P., Bryson, C., Purdon, S., Mallender, J., Bertranou, E., Jhita, T. and Roberts, S. (2013) *Evaluation of the Right to Control Trailblazers synthesis report*, London: DWP.

Tulle, E. and Dorrer, N. (2012) 'Back from the brink: ageing, exercise and health in a small gym', *Ageing and Society*, vol 32, no 7, pp 1106-27.

Twigg, J. (2006) *The body in health and social care*, Basingstoke: Palgrave.

Twigg, J. and Atkin, K. (1994) *Carers perceived: Policy and practice in informal care*, Milton Keynes: Open University Press.

Tyson, A. (2009) *Don't be fooled by the law: A report from In Control, following a conference held on 1 April, 2009*, London: In Control.

UNISON (2009) *Not waving but drowning: Paperwork and pressure in adult social work services*, London: UNISON.

UNISON (2011) *Stepping into the breach: Social work's paraprofessionals*, London: UNISON.

Venn, S. and Arber S. (2011) 'Daytime sleep and active ageing in later life', *Ageing and Society*, vol 31, no 2, pp 197-216.

Whittaker, K. (2011) 'Personalisation in a time of cuts', www. centreforwelfarereform.org/library/by-date/personalisation-in-a-time-of-cuts.html.

Williams C., Harris J., Hind T and Uppal S (2009) *Transforming adult social care: Access to information, advice and advocacy*, London: Putting People First, Improvement and Development Agency, Local Government Association.

Windle K., Wagland R., Forder J., D'Amico F., Janssen J. and Wistow G. (2009) *National evaluation of Partnerships for Older People Projects: Final report*, PSSRU Discussion Paper 2700, Canterbury: University of Kent.

Wood, C. and Grant, E. (2010) *Counting the cost*, London: Demos.

Woolham J. and Benton C. (2012) 'The costs and benefits of personal budgets for older people: evidence from a single local authority', *British Journal of Social Work*, pp 1-20, doi: 10.1093/bjsw/bcs086.

Yanow, D. (1996) *How does a policy mean? Interpreting policy and organizational actions*, Washington, DC: Georgetown University Press.

Yanow, D. (2000) *Conducting interpretive policy analysis*, London: Sage Publications.

Zarb, G. and Nadash, P. (1994) *Cashing in on independence: Comparing the costs and benefits of cash and services*, London: British Council of Organisations of Disabled People.

Index

Printed and bound by CPI Group (UK) Ltd, Croydon, CR0 4YY

27/10/2024

14580559-0002
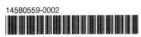